WATER WONDER WORKS TWO…

- manage pain
- strengthen muscles
- improve mobility

Exercise in the Comfort of Your Pool to Increase Your Range of Motion and Improve Overall Health

Marti C. Sprinkle

with Jennifer Sakauye, DPT
and Dan Steinberg, PT

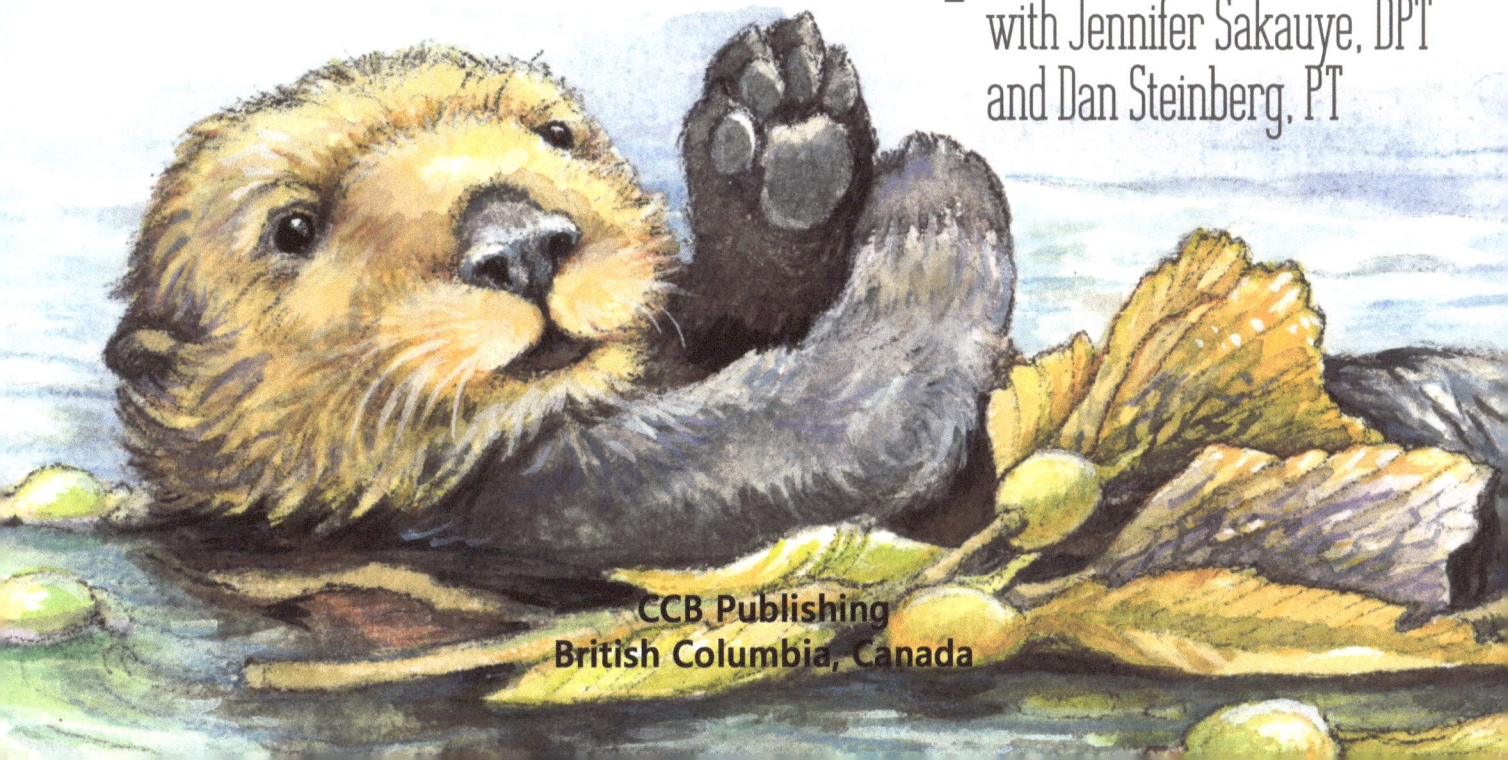

CCB Publishing
British Columbia, Canada

Water Wonder Works Two: Exercise in the Comfort of Your Pool to Increase Your Range of Motion and Improve Overall Health

Copyright ©2023 by Marti C. Sprinkle
ISBN-13 978-1-77143-560-4
First Edition

Library and Archives Canada Cataloguing in Publication
Sprinkle, Marti C., 1944-, author
Water wonder works two : exercise in the comfort of your pool to increase your range of motion and improve overall health / by Marti C. Sprinkle. – First edition.
Includes bibliographical references.
Issued in print and electronic formats.
ISBN 978-1-77143-559-8 (hbk.).--ISBN 978-1-77143-560-4 (pbk.).--ISBN 978-1-77143-561-1 (pdf)
Additional cataloguing data available from Library and Archives Canada

Photo credits: All photos contained herein are copyright Marti C. Sprinkle.
Cover design and section pages designed by: Susan Bateman, Graphic Designer

Publisher: CCB Publishing
               British Columbia, Canada
               www.ccbpublishing.com

Contents

Introduction

For quite some time my clients have requested a book of my exercises so that they could take the book with them when they traveled. Here it is.

Water Wonder Works Two features low-impact daily exercises, and an Introduction of Muscle Movements. Each section of the book has a pre-exercise statement page. The actions of the muscles impacted by the exercise are listed beneath each exercise. The exercises provide a total body workout.

Chapters begin with a warm-up followed by exercises for specific days of the week, ending with a cool down section. Finger and neck exercises are included within the weekly routine. A glossary of muscles for each area of movement can be found at the back of the book as can hand painted drawings showing the different muscles.

Self-selection of exercises to set up a water exercise routine or to strengthen a certain area of the body is possible using the exercises within this book. *Water Wonder Works Two* can become a personalized guide for individual routines. The exercises are designed to be used in any pool.

When performing a water aerobics exercise, it is difficult to determine which part of the body is involved because the whole body participates in the exercise. Unlike land exercises or weight machines, which isolate muscle or muscle groups, in water the total body becomes active with every exercise. Sometimes, one experiences pain, stress, or trauma to a certain muscle or muscle group. By selecting one or several of the exercises within this book, you can relieve the pain or muscle stress.

Water aerobics helps people who have had surgeries, strokes, Parkinson's disease, and joint replacements. It also helps cancer survivors regain confidence about their body, by developing more mobility and range of motion. Anyone can create an ability range of their own, using the exercises shown in this book. Some people may want to lose weight, but most will be strengthening muscles while developing a leaner body mass, and losing inches. Feeling better about oneself improves as does one's self-confidence.

Water aerobics promotes better overall health. Water is a miracle worker. May this book become a valuable tool as well as an asset, leading to a healthier lifestyle.

Acknowledgements

I especially wish to thank my clients for their support and loyalty. Testimonials throughout *Water Wonder Works Two* attest to how the exercises have helped their health.

I would like to express my gratitude to Bear Valley Springs, a non-profit corporation governing the resort community located in Tehachapi, California. Wesley Shryrock, MBA, CMCA, general manager and Debbie Papac, Bear Valley Springs recreation manager, allowed me to use the Oak Tree Country Club Pool for several photo shoots. In addition, I would also like to thank Sunny Olsen, BSc, manager of Evolutions Fitness and Wellness Center of Tulare Regional Health Care District, Tulare, California for the use of the pool during a brief photo shoot. Cameron West, Aquatic Integration Institute of Atascadero, California also let me use her home pool for a photo shoot.

My photographers did a wonderful job. Many thanks to Courtney Troffer, Just Another Shot Photography, Peter Faulks, and Michael McLane. Two of my models, Rusty and Malissa Wright assisted with photos using my Go-Pro camera.

I am immensely grateful to all the models who gave their time. A page with individual cameos and their fields of interest can be found near the back of *Water Wonder Works Two*.

I especially want to thank everyone who helped me edit this book for publication.

My daughter, Evelyn Sprinkle, Ph. BCBA-D, helped write my biography. It was great to have my number one fan club member help me in this regard.

My special friend and someone I consider an adopted daughter, graphic designer Susan Bateman, helped me with the design of the cover. She also helped design the sections pages. Thank you, Susan.

Leesa Greenlee, California Bay Area artist, hand painted the cover illustration and the front and back human body drawings. I am grateful to Leesa for her invaluable help.

Special thanks to all my instructors... Ruth Sova, Laurie Denomme, Terri Mitchell, Beth Scalone, and others... from the Aquatic Exercise and Rehabilitation Institute (ATRI) and the American Exercise Association (AEA). Many of their techniques added to my classes and inspired me.

Thanks and kudos to Kent and Karen Vaagen, proprietors of Steampunk Café and Grill where Dan Steinberg, PT and I spent many hours working on this book.

My computer technician, Greg Cunningham, tech-hachapi, a Microsoft certified technician, spent countless hours helping me line up photos and formatting the graphics on each page. His assistance was essential and most valuable towards the completion of *Water Wonder Works Two*.

With appreciation and additional thanks to South Street Digital, Inc. for editing and refining images to press quality condition.

Special Acknowledgements

I am grateful to <u>Daniel Steinberg</u>, BS, PT, MS and owner of Stone Mountain Physical Therapy, Tehachapi, California, for his invaluable help and encouragement with muscle and muscle groups mentioned within this book.

Dan Steinberg is a graduate of UC San Francisco Medical Center and received an advanced degree from UCLA. He taught at the University of New York, Buffalo and at Boston University. Dan has over 50 years of experience in the physical therapy field.

Many thanks to <u>Jennifer Sakauye</u>, DPT, who helped restructure this book. Jennifer received her BS degree in Physiological Science from UCLA. While attending UCLA, she participated in a three-year sports medicine internship. She devoted two of these years to Division I water polo athletes who had experienced acute injuries. Jennifer completed her Doctor of Physical Therapy degree at USC, where she earned a merit-based scholarship and an award in Foundational Sciences.

With a background in physics and physiology, Jennifer can identify body movements and target the forces acting upon muscles. She currently works at an aquatic and land-based physical therapy clinic in Culver City, California. Applying her knowledge of anatomy and biomechanics helps patients maximize their potential in the pool. Early years of competitive swimming gave Jennifer insight into the multiple benefits that water has upon the body.

This book is dedicated to Jay Sussell

and all my clients.

Explanation of Movement Analysis by Dan Steinberg, PT

Muscles are unique and important constituents of our body. A muscle has two functions: 1) provide stability to the skeletal system; and 2) move or cause movement of the skeletal system. A coordinated movement requires simultaneous action of the body's muscles to provide both stabilization and movement. Stability comes from an interaction between the body and an external force. Exercise cannot be performed or completed without stability and muscle movement.

Assumptions vary regarding the movement of muscles. These assumptions are related to the human body. The skeletal structure of the human body would collapse if not for the bone and joint structure and the ligaments and tendons holding it together. Ligaments attach bone to bone while tendons attach muscle to bone. The muscles of the skeletal structure pull from both ends to the middle of the muscle.

A muscle contraction can cause more than one bone to move at the same time. A two-joint muscle will move two adjacent bones by its tendons crossing over the two joints. Controlled movement occurs when the bone and muscle causing motion are stable, fixed or dynamically held stable.

Feet firmly placed upon the pool floor provide an external anchoring point for the body and stability to the legs. They transfer that stability by way of the bones and muscles to the torso, aligning with the pelvis. If the pelvis is stable, the torso will find stability and transfer that stability to the "shoulder girdle." The "shoulder girdle" is a complex area of the body made up of the clavicle (collar bone) attaching itself to the anterior chest wall at the sternum and to the scapula via the acromion. The scapula rests on the posterior chest wall, attaching the shoulder girdle to the torso. Because the shoulder is the source of arm movement, the humerus is included within the shoulder girdle with its attachment to the scapula. This complex area is held together by muscle and ligament tissue. This allows the "shoulder girdle" (glenohumeral joint) the greatest degree of movement of any joint in the musculoskeletal system. The integrity of this musculoskeletal complex is reliant on one small shallow joint as the only long point of skeletal stability. Therefore, the shoulder girdle is wholly reliant on the muscular-ligamentous system to maintain stability in the shoulder girdle while allowing the greatest freedom of movement.

Many of the exercises in this book involve grasping weights with the hands. There are two types of muscles that help achieve the grip. This is accomplished by muscles exclusively in the hand, called "intrinsic" muscles, and muscles that begin outside of the hand in the forearm but ultimately end in the hand, called Extrinsics. The Extensor Carpi Radialis Longus and Brevis muscles stabilize the wrist, which allows the Flexor Digitorum Superficialis and Profundis muscles to hold the weights with the help of the Interosseus muscles of the hand (Intrinsics).

My scientific analysis of pool exercises comes from over 50 years of observing and assessing human movement combined with data. The data comes from literature reviews, laboratory study, undergraduate and graduate studies of exercise.

These studies include and are not limited to exercise physiology, kinesiology and physical therapy. A major influence in my analytical skills comes from students in my kinesiology classes and laboratory patients whom I assessed and treated. My graduate study with Valerie Hunt, M.D. helped me observe the time, space, and force in human movement. I learned to acknowledge and correlate the movements to dimensions related to human behavior.

The Bibliography page recommends several books to complement this text: Anatomy, physiology of muscles, and analysis of movement known as Kinesiology can be found through reference materials.

WATER WONDER WORKS TWO...

is designed to provide low-impact exercises for all parts of the body. It is a practical approach to exercising. It can become a valuable asset to develop understanding of your body and lead to a healthier you.

Before using these exercises...

it is prudent to check with your physician if you have physical problems before taking a water aerobics class. If you are finishing physical therapy sessions, it is also advisable to check with your physical therapist before taking a class.

It is recommended NOT to do more than 15 minutes of a particular exercise motion at any given time. If an exercise causes muscle tension and becomes uncomfortable when performing it, be logical, and quit doing that particular exercise.

Common conditions to consider before getting into the water:

- open wounds
- skin conditions and scabies
- uncontrolled hypertension
- mental confusion
- menstruation cycle
- fever
- diarrhea
- effects of medications
- fear of water

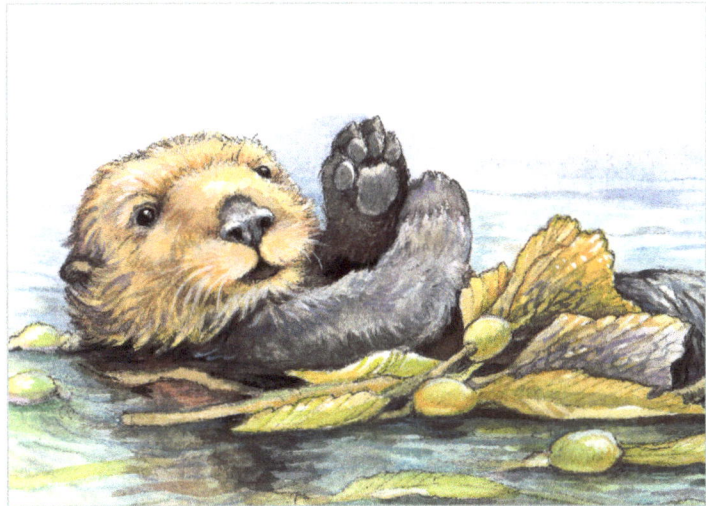

WARM UP

"About 5-6 years ago I began having pain in my left shoulder. My range of motion was limited. After seeking medical advice, and physical therapy, I decided to start Marti's water aerobics class. I was still experiencing pain. After taking the water classes for about a couple of months, three times a week, it occurred to me that my pain was gone, and I had regained my range of motion. To this day, I still have no pain in that shoulder and enjoy full range of motion. I credit Marti's water expertise with my full recovery." – Linda T.

Warm Up Pre-Exercise Muscle Information

Exercising in water lets you put full force on your joints without the effect of gravity. Water buoyancy cushions the joints, making exercising feel effortless. You are actually toning muscles more effectively than on land.

It is most important to warm up each area of your body.

Warming up increases oxygen and blood to the muscles being used, dilating blood vessels as circulation is increased. Warming up also increases body and muscle temperature. Hormones are released which allow fatty acids and carbohydrates to convert into energy for the muscle groups and the needed muscle activity.

Stretching the tendons and increasing circulation keeps your body limber, improves total body flexibility, and makes more difficult exercises easier. Warming up helps reduce muscle soreness. Less injury is sustained.

The exercises within the Warm Up section increase in intensity to the various muscle groups.

There are several different types of muscle contractions addressed in this book:

- Isometric muscle contraction: There is no movement at the joint. The main part of the muscle, the belly, is tightening but no movement occurs. The Trapezius muscles stabilize the scapula is an example. The muscle contracts but no movement occurs.

- Concentric muscle contraction: There is movement at the joints. The muscle belly is tightening, or "balling up", causing a movement by pulling on the least stable bone. The muscle is shortening.

- Eccentric muscle contraction: There is movement at the joint, but it is occurring because of the "balled up" muscle "letting go" under control. The muscle lengthens. Ex: The "letting go" of the Biceps on the arm when the forearm slowly lowers a heavy weight away from the torso. This action is used when slowly controlling the weight to "pop up" to the surface of the water.

Jogging

Between each exercise I recommend that a person jog to keep up their circulation. There are a few exercises to which this will not apply such as the slower ones that involve back stretching and the ones used for a cool down.

When jogging the person uses small steps in place bringing up the knees as high as personally desired. However, it is best to elevate the knee as much as possible so the knee joint becomes bent and moved, and the hip joint is activated.

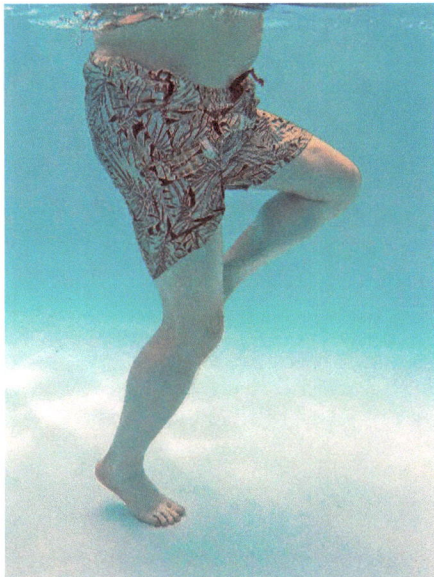

The person uses small steps, flat feet or on the ball of the foot, like a simulated running in place. The knee is flexed and moved upward as high a personally desired. The hip joint becomes activated.

ACTION: Jogging recruits Ankle Plantar flexors, Gastrocnemius and Soleus group of muscles, hip flexors on the Iliopsoas, pelvic stabilizers, and the Quadratus Lamborium.

The transverse abdominals and Multifictus help stabilize the torso as the leg is elevated. These same muscles engage for the lifting of the leg; straighten the knee engages the Gluteus Maximus at the hip, the Quadriceps at the knee, and the Gastrocnemius and Soleus at the ankle.

Big Arm Circles

Helps increase mobility of the arms, shoulders, and upper torso.

The water should be shoulder height for the best execution of this exercise.

Bring both arms to the surface of the water, holding the weights. Extend the arms out to the side as far as possible. Keep the arms in line with the shoulders as palms are facing forward while holding the weights.

Pull the weights down and in toward the chest, bending the elbows. Keep the weights close to the surface of the water. Continue the inward motion toward the chest. Return the hands with the weights to the original position, in line with the shoulders.

Repeat this movement 20 to 25 times.

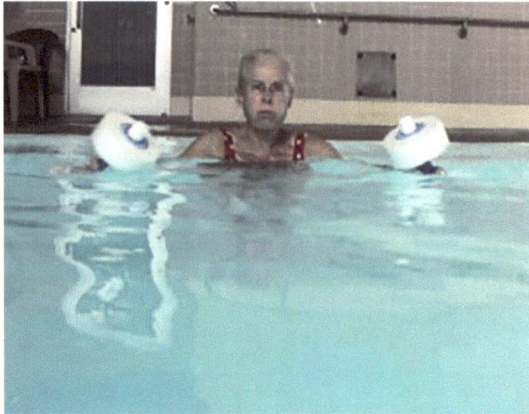

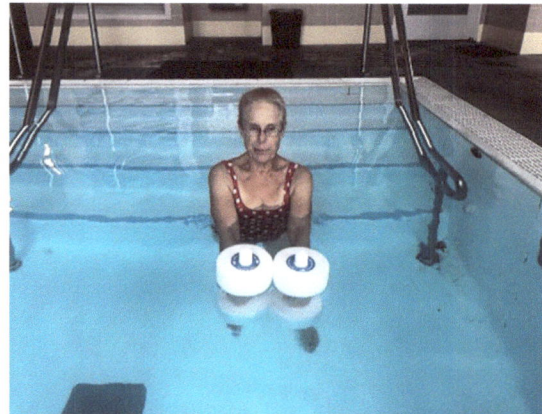

ACTION: The buoyancy of the water holds the arms in front of the body and along the surface of the water. The movement involved in this exercise is horizontal abduction and scapular retraction when moving the arms out and horizontal adduction to bring the arms back to the center (see glossary for muscles that perform these motions).

Flying

Helps increase mobility of the upper torso, arms, and neck. Increases flexibility.

Place arms out at the sides; hold weights with palms down. Keep arms at shoulder height.

Keeping the arms straight, move them down and up as if flying. The arms should move down and up about 6 to 8 inches below the water's surface. Return the weights to the water's surface after each "flying" movement.

Repeat "flying" movement 20 to 25 times.

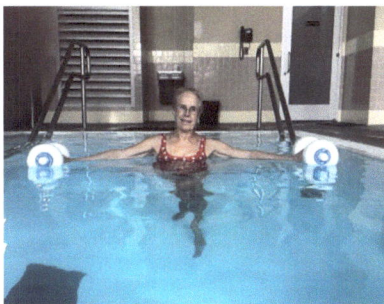

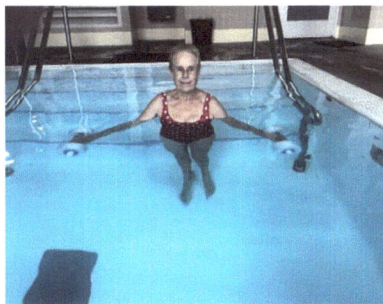

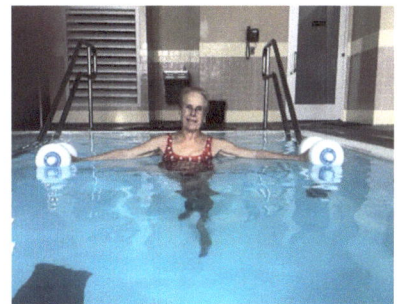

ACTION: Pulling the arms down to the hips is a concentric contraction of the shoulder adductors. Slowly controlling the arms back up so they don't "pop up" to the surface of the water is an eccentric contraction of the same muscles. Holding the arms straight and palms down requires isometric contractions of the elbow extensors and forearm pronators (exact muscles listed in glossary).

Left Arm/Right Arm

Helps increase mobility in the shoulders, arms, neck, and upper torso. Stretches upper torso and lateral (side) abdominal muscles.

Hold arms are in front of the torso with the weights held vertically. Thumbs should be up.

The left arm stays straight in front of the torso. Move the right arm out to the right side even with the shoulder. The right arm returns to the front of the torso into the original position. Repeat this right arm movement 12 to 15 times.

The right arm stays still in front of the torso. Move the left arm out to the left side, even with the left shoulder. Return the left arm to the front of the torso into the original position. Repeat this left arm movement 12 to 15 times.

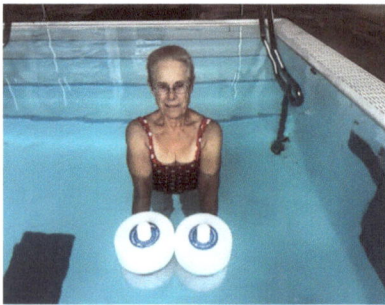

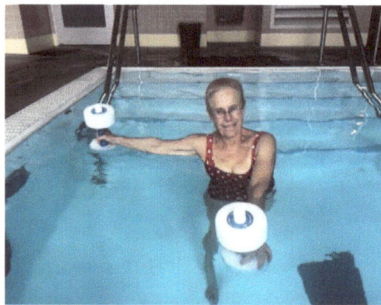

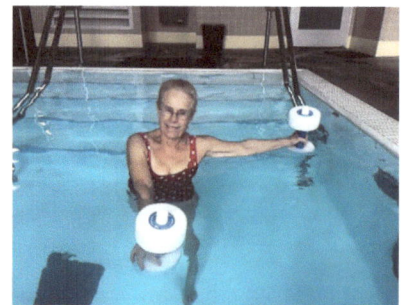

ACTION: The outward movement of the arm is horizontal abduction and scapular retraction. Bringing the arm back to the center is horizontal adduction and scapular protraction. An isometric abdominal contraction is necessary here to keep the trunk stable and avoid leaning to either side when the arms move.

Jog Punching

Helps increase stamina, balance, spinal alignment, and circulation.

Jog Punching #1 – While jogging in place, push one weight down by the hip. As you raise that weight push the other one down. Repeat 20 to 25 times.

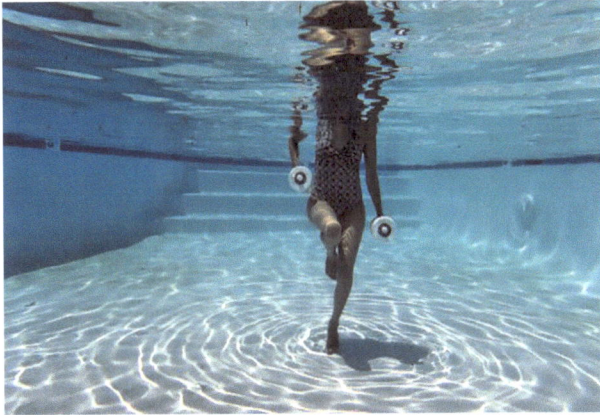

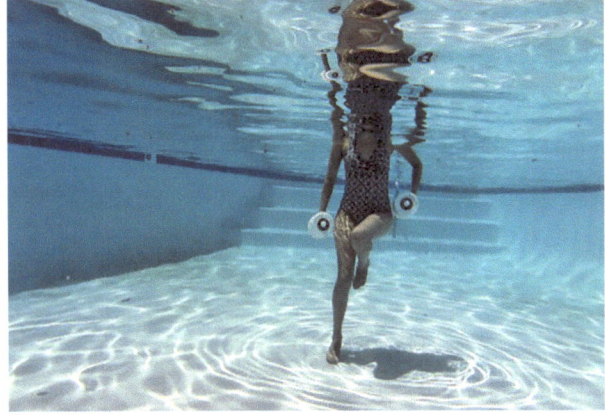

Jog Punching #2 - Push the weights in front of your body alternating sides and making sure your elbows are pulled backward and as close to the torso as possible, waist high.

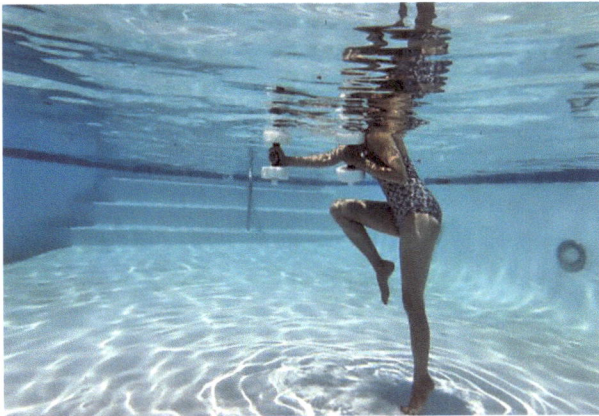

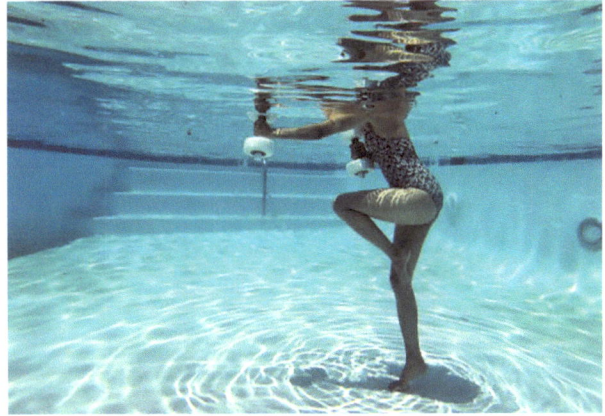

ACTION: Lifting the leg involves hip flexion, knee flexion and ankle plantarflexion while pushing it back down to the ground involves hip extension, knee extension and ankle dorsiflexion. The arm movements for jog punching #1 and #2 are achieved by alternating contractions of the shoulder flexors and elbow extensors and shoulder extensors and elbow flexors. Jog punching #1 will force a greater contraction of these muscles as you are pushing straight down against the water buoyancy.

Jog Punching #3 - Push both weights forward and then pull both weights inward toward the torso. Make sure the elbows are bent and close to the torso, waist high.

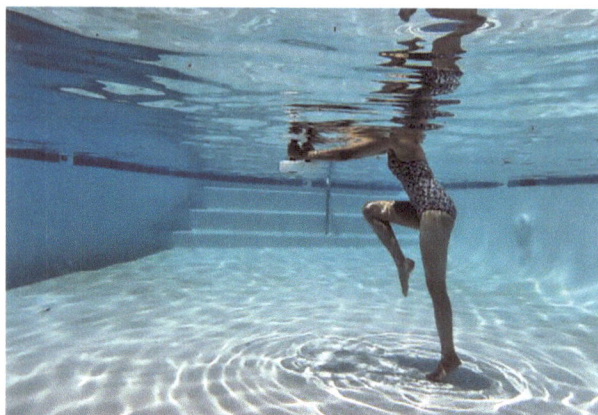

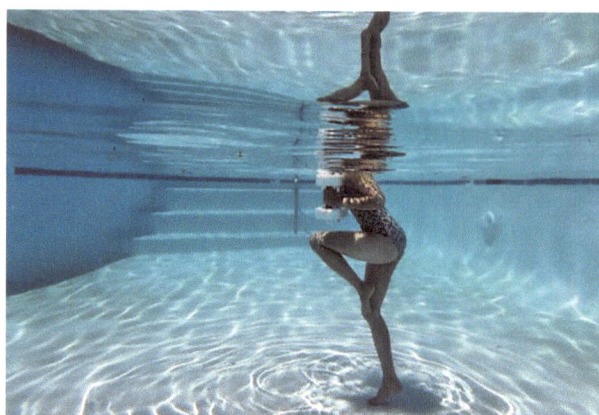

Jog Punching #4 - Push the weights downward alternating from right to left. As the left knee comes upward during the jog, push the right weight downward to touch the top of the right knee or thigh as it moves across the torso. As the right knee comes upward during the jog, the left weight pushes downward to touch the top of the left knee or thigh moving it across the torso.

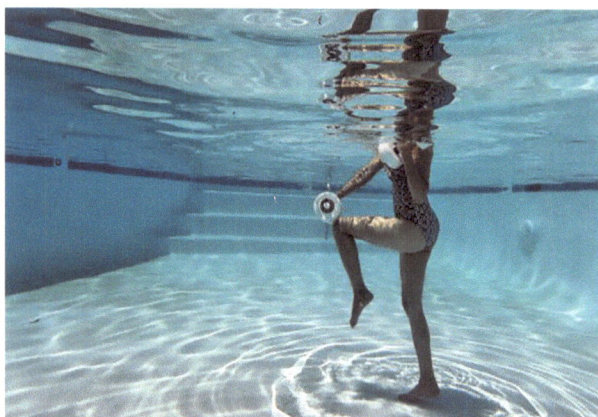

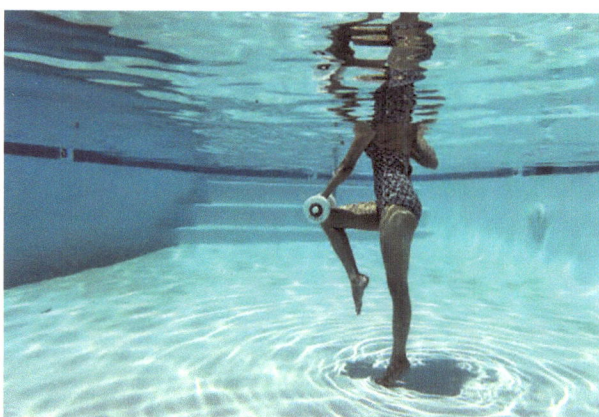

ACTION: The same lower extremity muscles are used for jogging. Jog punching #3 will use the shoulder flexors and elbow extensors to push the weights in front of the body, and the shoulder extensors and elbow flexors to pull the weights inward. Jog punching #4 utilizes the same arm muscles in an alternating pattern and involves trunk rotation to help strengthen the abdominals (exact muscles listed in glossary).

Jumping Jacks
(Half Jacks in the Water)

Helps improve balance, coordination, arm, and leg strength. Stretches and strengthens arms legs, and abdominal muscles.

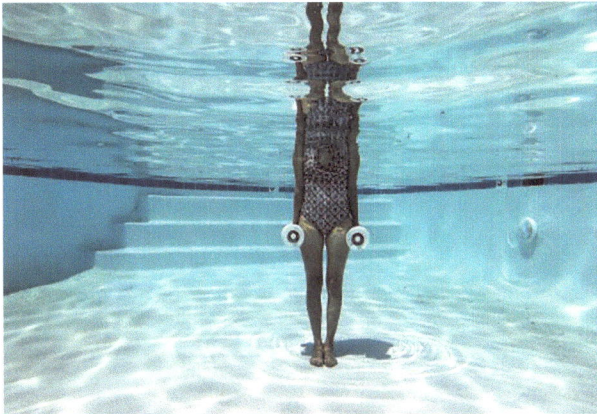

Pull the weights to the sides of the torso at the thighs, keeping palms inward and down at the sides. Arms are held straight at the torso next to the thighs. The legs should be held together. Jump and move the arms out to the side as the jump is completed (see direction below).

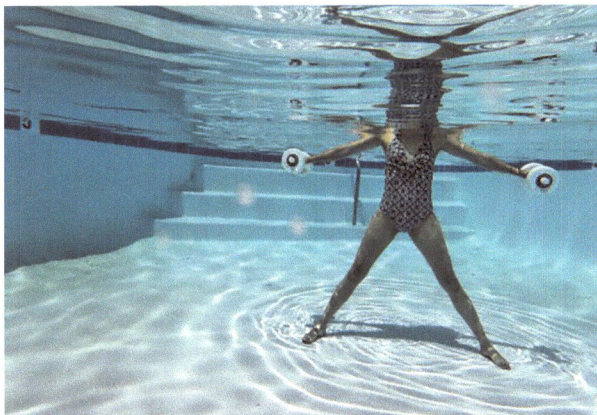

Raise the arms upward from the thighs to the water's surface, as the legs move outward in a jumping motion. Legs should form a capital letter A. Jump back inward to the starting position. Return the legs and arms to their original position, with both arms to the sides and legs together.

Repeat this outward and back inward movement of the arms and legs 25 times.

ACTION: Jumping requires a quick contraction of the hip extensors, knee extensors and ankle plantar flexors to generate force off the ground. Pushing the legs out to the side is achieved with a concentric contraction of the hip abductors and raising the arms is an eccentric contraction of the shoulder adductors. To control the landing, the body performs an eccentric contraction of the same lower extremity muscles used to jump and the arms are pulled back to the sides with the shoulder adductors.

Cross Over Jumping Jacks
(Half Jacks in the Water with a Leg Crossover)

Helps improves balance, coordination, pelvic stability, and alignment.

Holds weights with palms down and pull them downward to the side of the torso to touch the thighs.

Raise the arms at the same time as the legs move outward to make a large capital letter A.

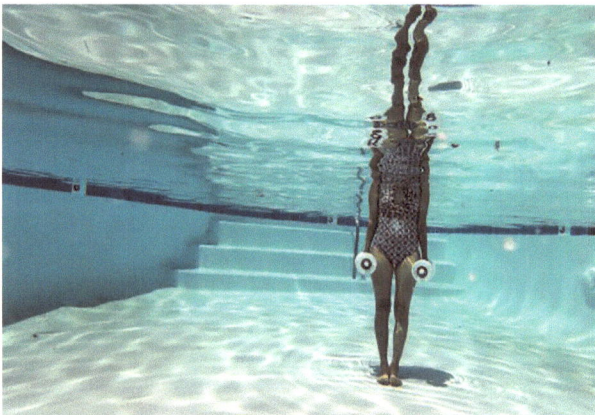

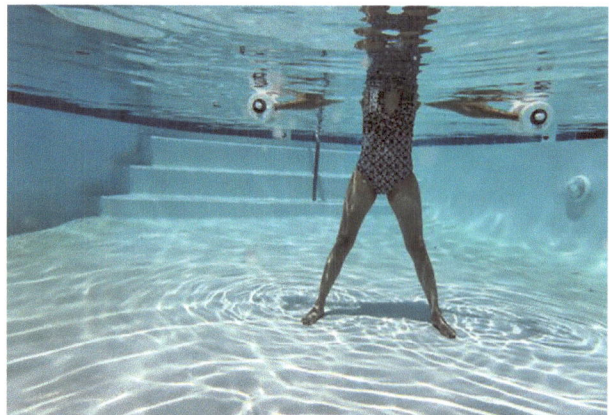

Cross the left leg over the right leg as the legs come together.

Repeat this cross over scissor movement with the jumping jack arms and leg 25 times.

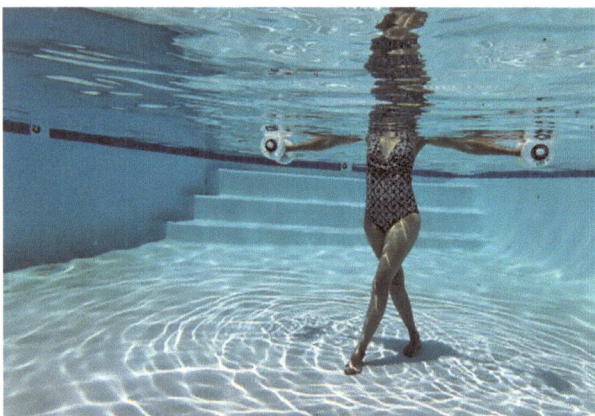

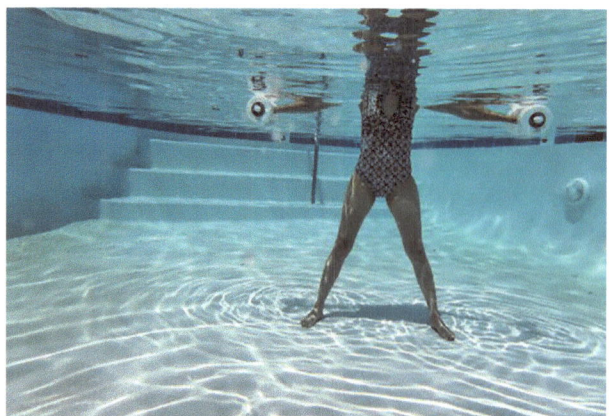

Photo above shows arms at shoulder height for a better view of leg positions.

ACTION: This exercise uses the same muscles as the jumping jacks but with greater activation of the hip adductors with the crossover.

High Intensity Interval Training Style Jumping Jacks
(A Variation of the Jumping Jacks Exercise)

Helps strengthen and stretch upper shoulders and upper back.

Hold the weights vertically in front of the torso with straight arms.

Move the legs and arms out at the same time, like the jumping jack's exercise. Legs form a capital letter A; straight arms are in line with the shoulders slightly below the surface of the water. Move straight arms and legs out and back to original position 25 times.

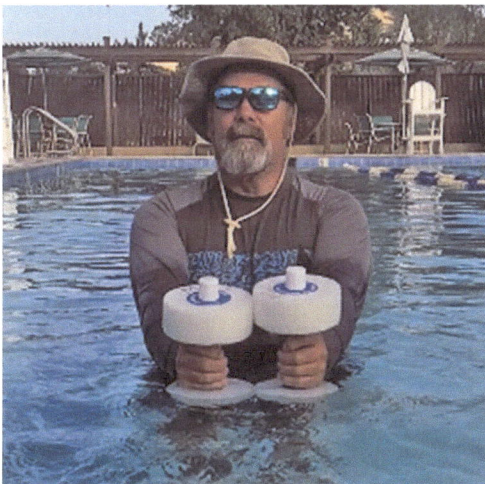

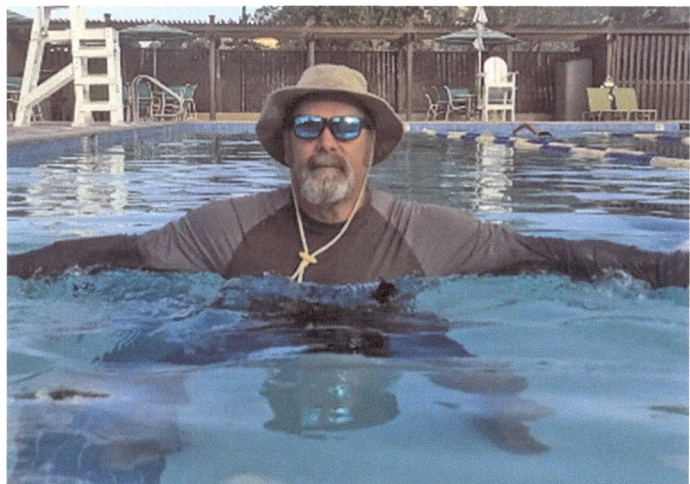

ACTION: This exercise uses the same lower extremity muscles as the jumping jacks to perform the quick jump and soft landing. The arm motion uses the shoulder horizontal abductors to bring them out to the side and the shoulder horizontal adductors to bring them back to the center (exact muscles listed in the glossary).

Rocking Horse

Helps improve balance, flexibility, coordination, and back strength.

The photos below show the arms out to the side, and exaggerated leg movement.

The weights are held, palms down. Elbows should be bent near the chest and at the water's surface, slightly in front and lower than the shoulders. Place the right foot in front of the left foot and bend the knees slightly.

Shift the body forward to the right foot and back again to the left foot which should come slightly off the pool floor. Repeat this "rocking" motion 25 times with the right foot forward.

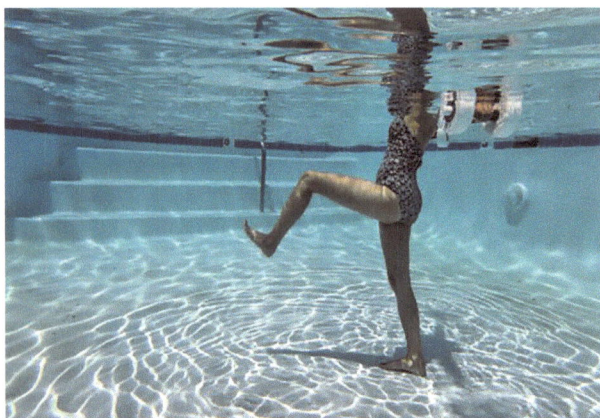

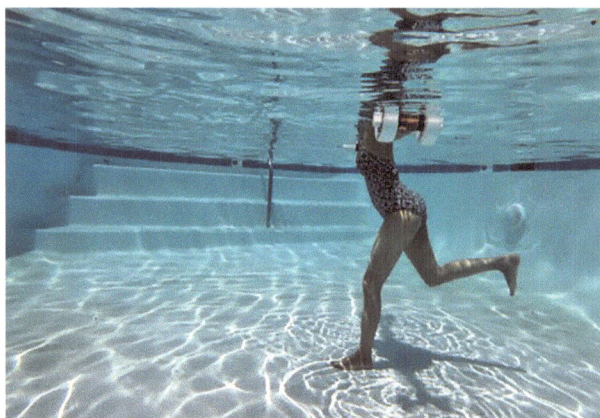

Then, switch feet, placing the left foot in front of the right as the knees bend slightly. The person shifts their body forward to the left foot and back again to the right foot which should come slightly off the pool floor. Repeat the "rocking" movement 25 times with the left foot forward.

This exercise may be intensified by rowing with the "weighted" hands as the torso is shifted forward/backward.

ACTION: Jumping forward onto the left leg requires a quick contraction of the right hip extensors, knee extensors and ankle plantar flexors. Receiving the body's weight onto the left leg uses these same muscles in an eccentric contraction to slow the body's descent. Shifting the body weight forward requires contraction of the abdominals and shifting it back activates the back extensors (muscles listed in glossary).

Can-Can

Helps improve range of motion, balance, coordination, hip, and body strength.

Both feet are on the pool floor. The person hops on the left foot and pulls up the right knee. The right leg is then straightened and pulled down with the heel. The person then hops on the right foot, pulling up the left knee. The left leg is straightened and pulled down with the heel. The leg movement is an alternating movement between right/left and is repeated for 25 times.

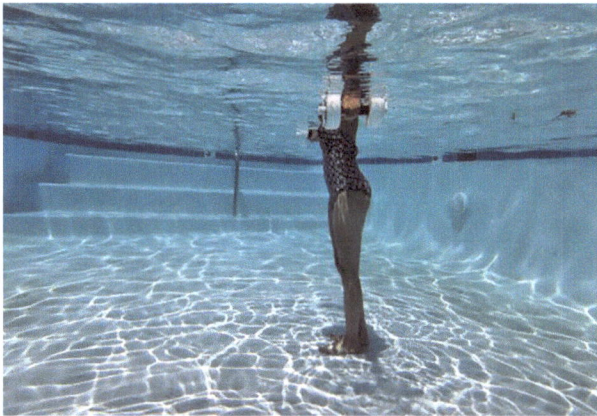

Both feet are on the pool floor.

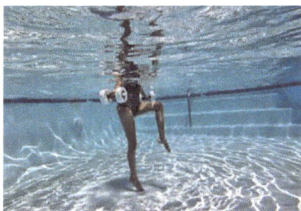

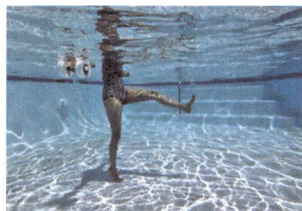

The person hops on the right foot, pulling up the left knee. The left leg is then straightened and pulled down with the heel.

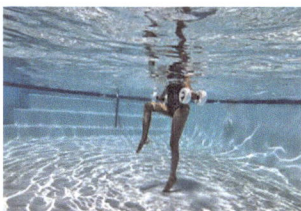

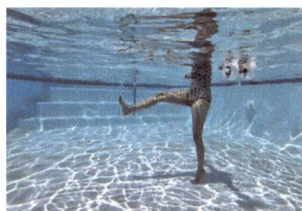

The person hops on the left foot, pulling up the right knee. The right leg is then straightened and pulled down with the heel.

The alternating leg movement between right/left is repeated for 25 times.

ACTION: The Hop: "Setting the Spring" is a lengthening (concentric) contraction of the Gluteus Maximus at the hip, Quadriceps at the knee, and Gastrocnemius at the ankle. This movement is followed by a concentric contraction of the knee by the same muscles for the left portion of the hop.

The thigh movement engages the Iliopsoas muscle. The kick at the knee then engages the Quadriceps muscle. The Gluteus Maximus draws the straightened leg down to the pool floor.

13

Snow Skiing... Moguls

(Hopping with Both Feet Together from Side-to-Side)

Helps improves balance, coordination, dexterity, motor skills, lower body muscles, and overall strength.

This exercise begins with knees and ankles together. One slightly bends the knees and hops to first the ride side and then, the left side as if jumping across a line in the pool or a mogul.

This hopping from right to left is repeated for 25 times.

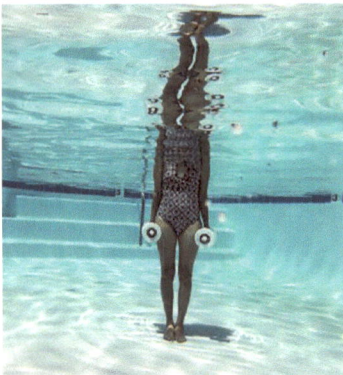

This exercise begins with knees and ankles together.

ACTION: This action is an isometric (holding) contraction of the Adductor longus and Magnus muscles.

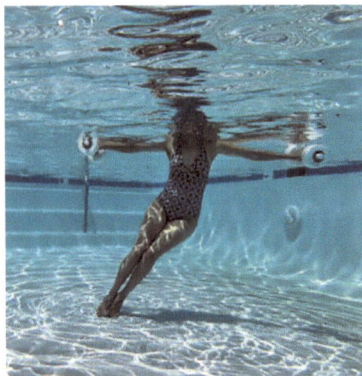

One slightly bends the knees and hops to first the right side as if jumping across a line in the pool or a mogul while snow skiing.

ACTION: This movement is a lengthening (eccentric contraction) of the Quadriceps muscles followed by a shortening (concentric contraction) of the same muscles along with the ankle plantar flexors: the Gastrocnemius, Tibialis Posterior, and Soleus muscles.

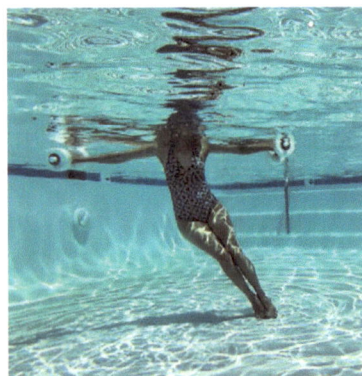

One slightly bends the knees and hops to the left side as if jumping across a line in the pool or a mogul when snow skiing. The hopping from side to side is repeated for 25 times. One hop to the right and one hop to the left constitutes one time.

The Twist, Side-to-Side

Helps improve mobility, balance, knee, and foot movement. Stretches lateral (side) abdominal muscles.

The knees and ankles are together as in the previous exercise (Snow Skiing). The person keep the heels planted on the pool bottom as the forefoot is alternately rotated to the left and then to the right. The person rapidly turns both toes to the right and then to the left with a twisting motion. Turning both feet first to the right and then to the left is counted as one time. This twisting is repeated for 25 times.

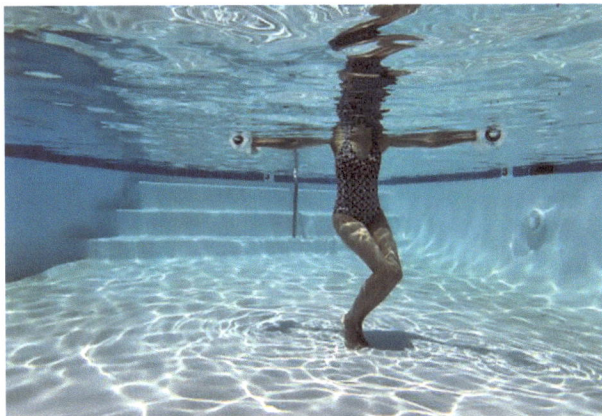

The knees and ankles are together as in the previous exercise. The person keep the heels planted on the pool bottom as the forefoot is alternately rotated to the left and then to the right.

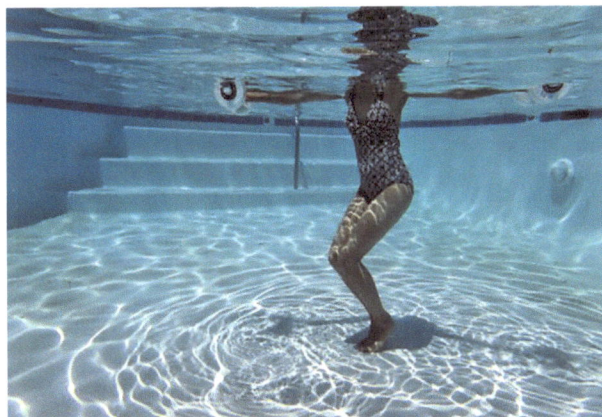

ACTION: The action of rotating the forefoot inward is an inversion and outward is an eversion. Inversion is the action of the Peroneus Longus, Brevis and Tertius muscles. The Anterior Tibalis, and Posterior Tibalis invert the forefoot.

Double Hops with Both Feet

Helps improve balance, mobility, and endurance. Increases agility.

Hold knees and ankles together.

Hop forward; then, backward, to the left and then to the right. Hop once in each direction. A hop in each of the four directions is considered one set. Repeat hopping motion 20 times.

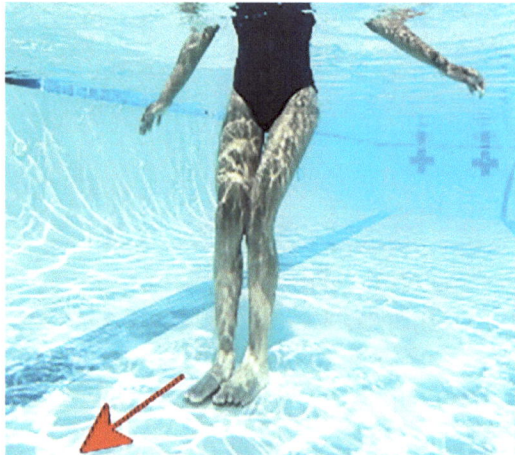

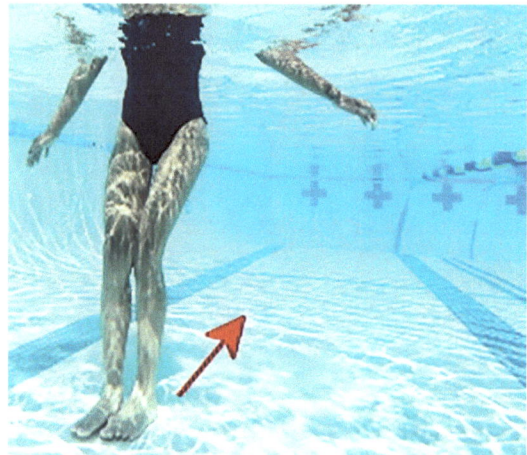

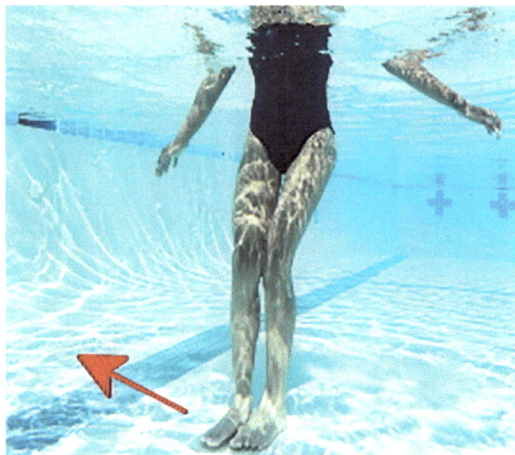

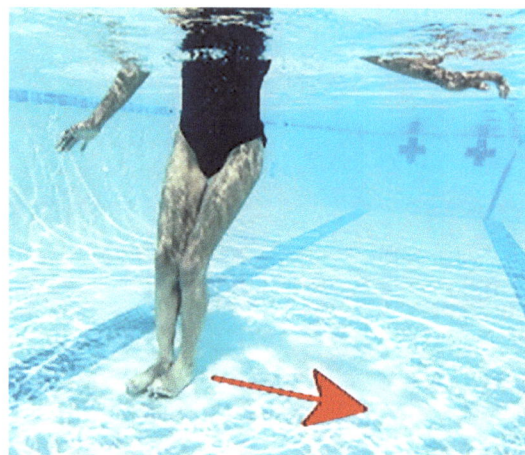

ACTION: Holding the knees and ankles together is an isometric contraction of the hip adductors. Hopping forwards and backwards activates the hip extensors, knee extensors, and ankle plantar flexors. This also requires activation of the trunk flexors and extensors. Hopping side to side requires the same muscles as above with additional activation of the hip abductors and adductors. The trunk side bend muscles must be used to stabilize the body in the sideways hopping.

Stomping Grapes

Helps hips, flexibility, balance, and coordination. Strengthens arms, shoulders, and legs.

The weights are held out to the side of the torso near the water's surface. Feet are turned outward facing the weights, making a large capital letter A position. Knees are bent as close to a 90-degree angle as possible.

Pull alternating knees up and down/left and right foot (stomping grapes) for 25 stomps on each foot. Each left/right stomp is counted as one stomp.

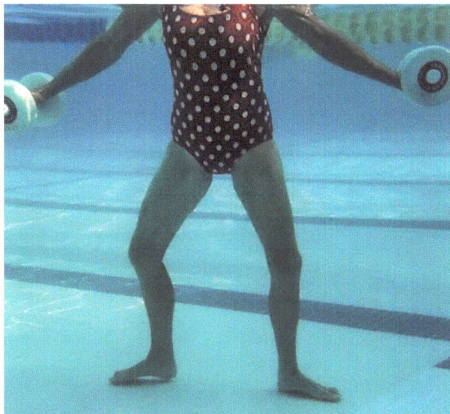

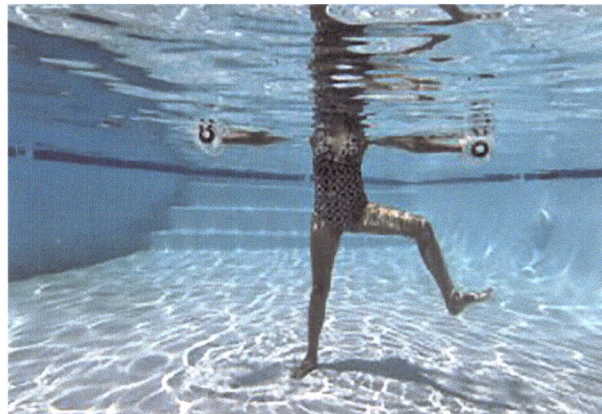

Continue to stomp, pull weights inward and bring them together mid-torso in front of the hips. Then, return the arms return to their original position. The weights are pulled inward/outward 25 times.

Stop the arm movement and continue to stomp, right and left 25 additional times.

ACTION: Obtaining the starting position uses the hip external rotators and knee flexors. Lifting the leg uses the hip abductors and flexors while the standing leg must use the hip extensors, knee extensors and ankle plantar flexors to stabilize the legs and the body.

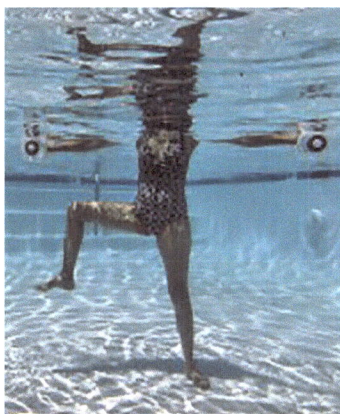

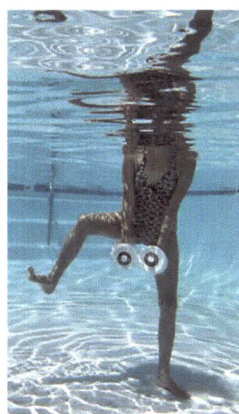

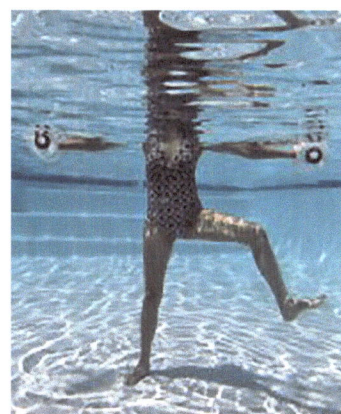

ACTION: Pulling the arms in front of the torso with palms facing down utilizes the shoulder adductors and forearm pronators.

Nordic Skier

Helps flexibility, coordination, and balance. Strengthens knees, pelvic and lower body muscles.

Hold weights vertically with the palms inward. The left leg scissors or slides forward. The right arm moves/pushes forward with the same movement as the left leg. The right arm pulls backward toward the chest area as the leg moves backwards like walking.

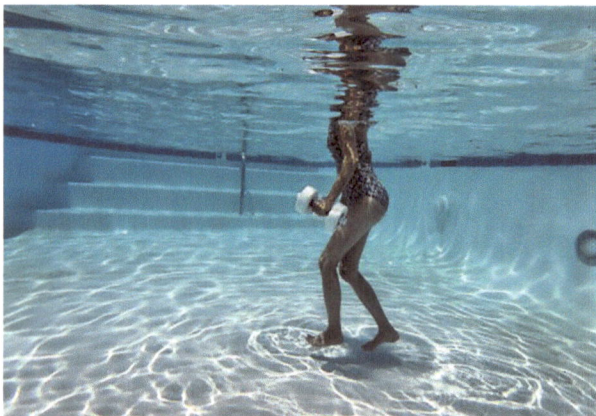

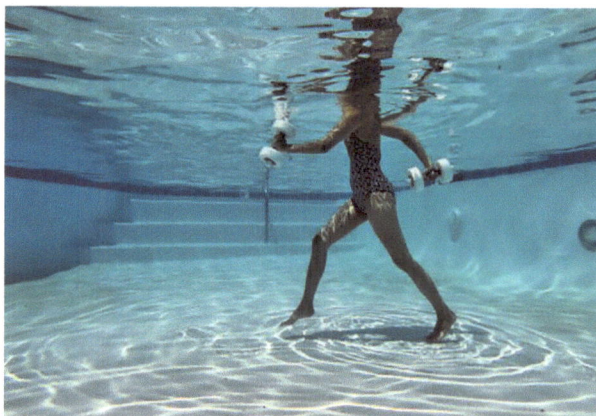

The right leg scissors or slides forward. The left arm moves/pushes forward with the same movement as the right leg. The left arm pulls backward toward the chest area as the leg moves backwards, like walking.

The forward movement of the right leg and then the left leg, arms moving opposite the legs, is one repetition. Repeat 40 times.

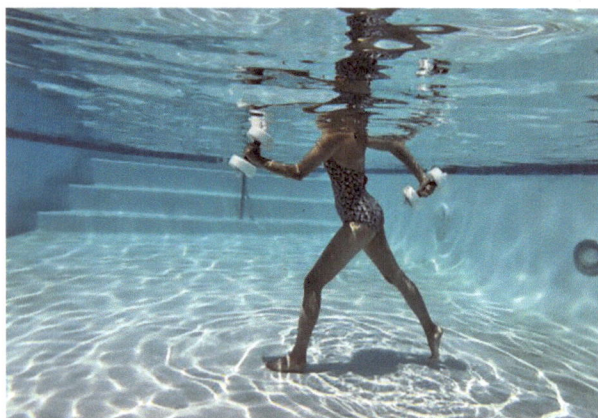

ACTION: Forward movement of the leg utilizes the hip flexors and knee extensors while backwards movement of the leg uses the hip extensors and knee flexors. Moving the arm forward with the weight activates the shoulder flexors and moving them backwards activates the shoulder extensors. An eccentric contraction of the shoulder extensors is required to slow the arm from popping out of the water in front of the body and an eccentric contraction of the shoulder flexors keeps it from popping out of the water behind the body.

Running in Place
(Feet Off of the Pool Floor)

Helps balance, shoulder strength, improves lower body movement and supports cardio.

Hold the weights with palms down. Bend the elbows and push the weights down close to the hips and in line with the torso.

The straight arms continue to be held in place near and close to the hips throughout the exercise. Bend knees bend and pull feet upward and off the pool floor.

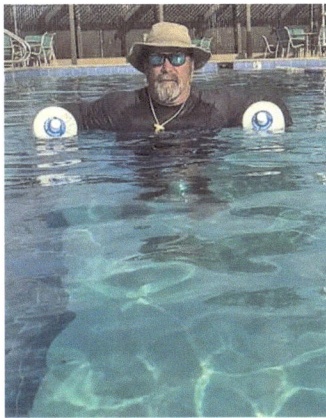

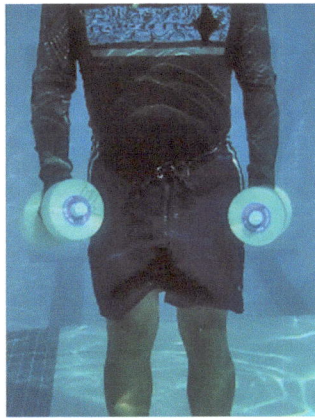

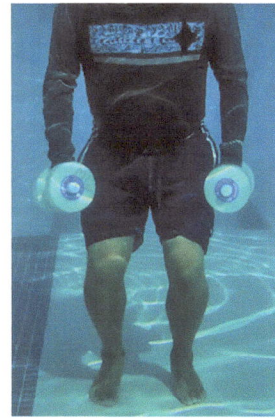

Arms are kept straight and close to the hips as you run in place with feet off the pool floor. Keeping the back straight with good posture helps the execution of this exercise. Run in place with arms close to the hips 30 to 40 seconds, or by individual counts to 30 or 40.

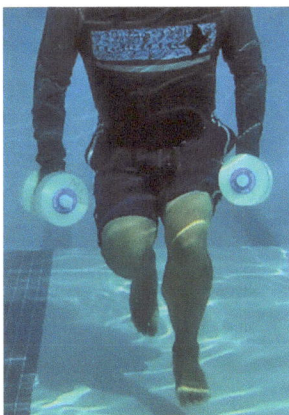

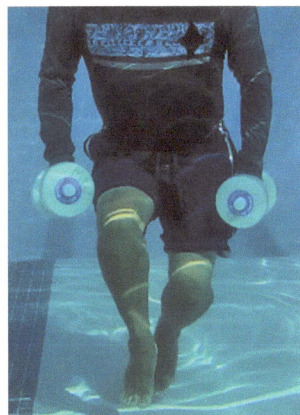

ACTION: Pushing the arms down under water to float the body utilizes the shoulder extensors, elbow flexors and trunk flexors to stabilize the body. Lifting the leg forwards activates the hip flexors while pushing the leg back uses the hip extensors. Keeping the knees bent the entire time is an isometric contraction of the knee flexors.

Front/Back Scissor Kicking
(Feet Off of the Pool Floor)

Helps coordination, balance, flexibility, and strengthens arms and legs.

Continue to hold the weights near the hips as in the previous exercise. Then move legs in a front-to-back scissor kick with the feet off the pool floor.

The right leg pushes forward/left weight pulls back as the left weight moves forward to maintain balance to the right side of the body.

Then, as the left leg pushes forward/right weight pulls backward, move the right weight forward to maintain balance.

Complete scissor kick with the feet off the pool floor 25 times. One right leg/one left leg counts as one repetition.

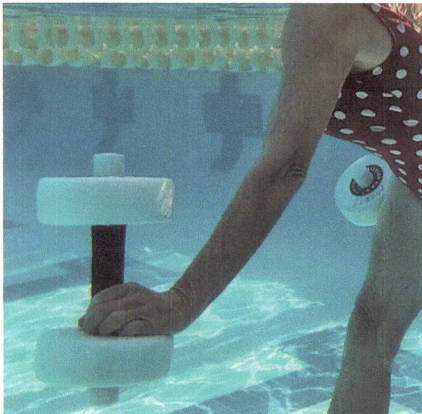

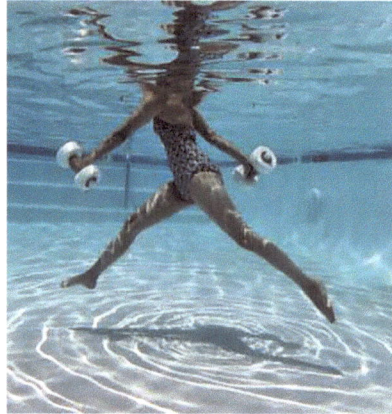

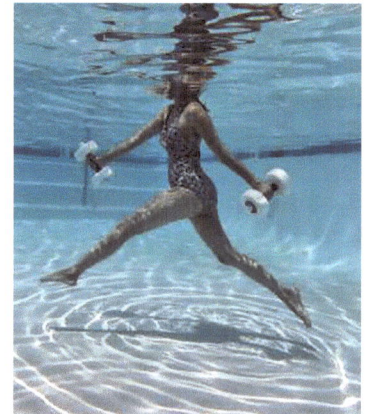

Photo #1 shows hand placement on the weight.

ACTION: The hand position for this exercise utilizes the wrist flexors and ulnar deviators to resist the water buoyancy pulling the weights to the surface. Keeping the leg straight and the toe pointed is an isometric contraction of the knee extensors and ankle plantar flexors. Bringing the leg forwards activates the hip flexors while kicking it backwards utilizes the hip extensors.

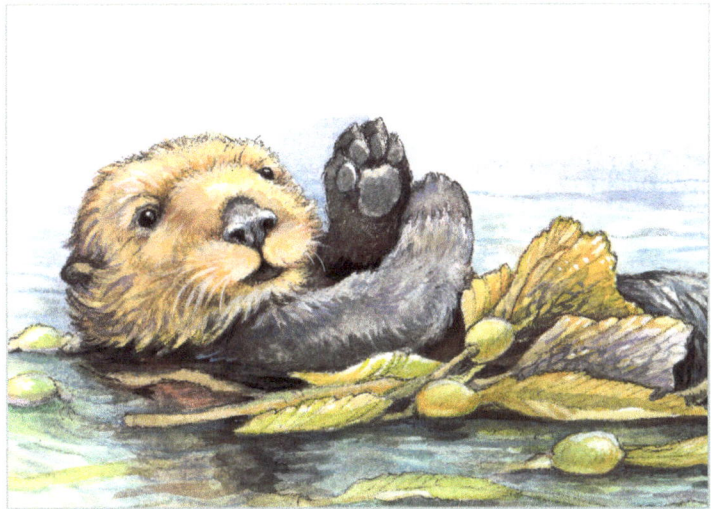

FINGERS

"Water aerobics is the best workout ever!
It keeps me strong, toned and healthy.
My spirit is lifted daily as we enjoy the great
outdoors, peppy music, and an instructor who
really knows her stuff. Water aerobics has
become an obsession with me. It's my way of
staying fit." – Wanda F.

Fingers Pre-Exercise Muscle Information

NOTE: Placing the weights under the armpits can be a problem with circulation. They should be used like a flotation device for the arms, or placed in a crossed position in front of the torso and not used at all.

Your hands are full of muscles and always in constant motion. Hands can suffer the same injuries as other parts of your body. It is very important to keep the fingers and hands stretched to combat aching, soreness, and arthritis in the hands. Keeping the fingers and thumbs limber restores range of motion to the fingers and wrists, improving the flow of blood to the hands. Flexible fingers can improve typing, and computer skills. Activities of daily living such as brushing teeth, putting on clothing, and lifting can be improved as the fingers and hands become stronger. One of the largest and most used appendages of your body is the thumb. Arthritis often begins at the thumb joint.

The exercises within this section are intended to improve range of motion and increase flexibility while strengthening hand performance.

The photos in this section come from my earlier book *Water Wonder Works... A Guide To Therapeutic Exercises*. These photos show more detailed movements.

The forearm position, supinated or pronated, gives a sense of muscle tension and effort. Pronation refers to the forearm position when the palm is facing down towards the floor. Supination is the forearm position when the palm is face up. Author's opinion: The prone/pronated fans are assisted with stabilization by the pronators of the wrist on the palmar surface of the forearm. Supinated fans are assisted with stabilization of the Supinators of the wrist on the dorsal surface of the forearm.

Finger "Fans" (Palms Down)

Helps flexibility of fingers, strengthens hands, and helps keep arthritis at bay.

The palms are held down and flat, on the surface of the water. Fingers are brought together. Spread the fingers outward, making a fan shape, and then bring them back together. Repeat "fan" shape 12 to 25 times.

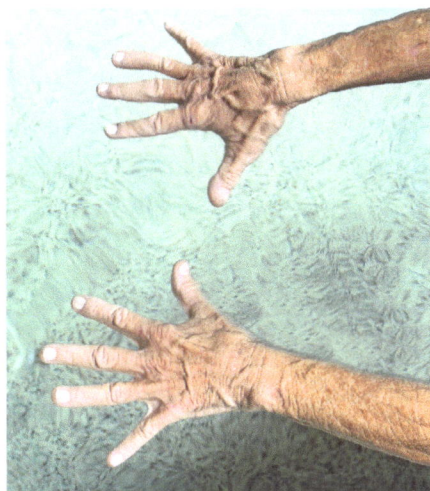

ACTION: Keeping the palms down requires activation of the forearm pronators. Spreading the fingers outwards is finger abduction and bringing them back together is finger adduction. The fingers are spread apart and brought back together by a combination action of the palmar and dorsal Interossei muscles.

Finger Fists (Palms Down)

Helps dexterity of the fingers, strengthens wrists and hands.

The fingers are held together and the palms down and flat, or prone to the surface of the water in front of the torso. The fingers of both hands make a fist and release while thrusting the fingers forward and then fisting them again. The thumb stays under the knuckles of the fisted fingers. Repeat fist and release motion 12 to 25 times.

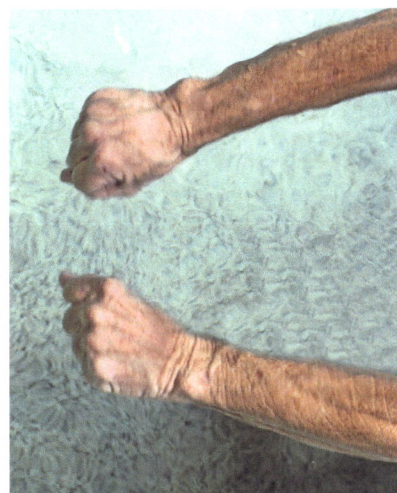

ACTION: Holding the palms down activates the forearm pronators and making a fist uses the intrinsic muscles in the palmar aspect of the hands. Straightening the fingers back out uses the muscles in the dorsal part of the hands.

Finger "Fans" (Palms Up)

Helps strengthen the hands, stretches tendons increasing flexibility.

Hold fingers together, with flat palms facing upward. Spread fingers of both hands out to the sides, like a fan, and return them to their original position. Repeat "fanning" action 12 to 25 times.

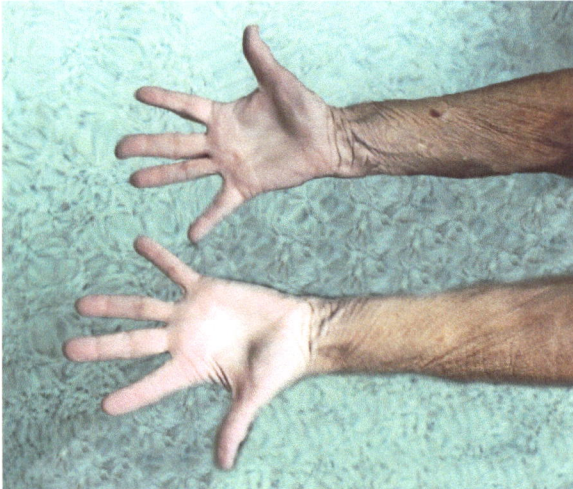

ACTION: This exercise uses the same muscles as the other finger fan exercise but due to the palms up position, it activates the forearm supinators.

Finger Fists (Palms Up)

Helps with grasping objects, strengthens hands and fingers.

Hold fingers together. Flat palms are held upward, floating on the water's surface. The fingers of both hands are then "fisted" and thrust open. The fingers are then returned to a fisted position. Repeat fisting and releasing action of the fingers 12 to 25 times.

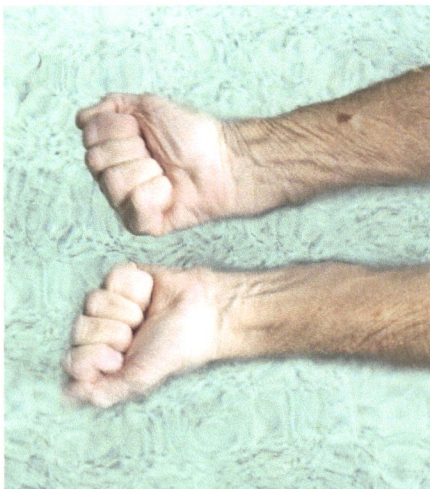

ACTION: This exercise uses the same muscles as the previous finger fist exercises, but due to the palms up position, it activates the forearm supinators.

Piano

Helps finger flexibility, stretches tendons in the hands.

Hold the palms down and hands flat and parallel to the surface of the water, with fingers extended and slightly separated. Pull each finger down separately, both hands at the same time. Begin the "piano" playing moving from the thumbs to the pinkie and back. Repeat this movement of "piano" playing approximately 12 times.

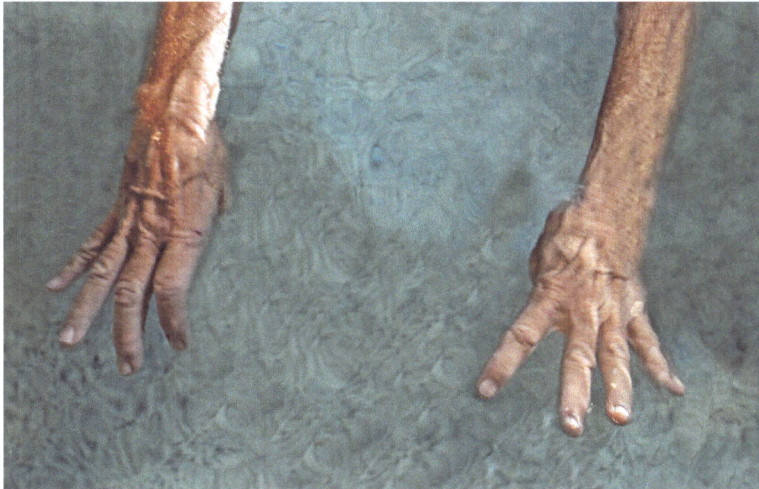

ACTION: Holding the palms down and spreading the fingers utilizes the forearm pronators and dorsal interossei muscles of the hand. Pulling each finger down engages the flexor digitorum superficialis muscle, an interior compartment of the forearm.

Claw Like a Cat

Helps strengthen finger knuckles, wrists, and lower arms.

Both hands are held in front of the torso in a relaxed position slightly below the water's surface. The fingers are moved in a clawing motion to the first knuckles. Then, the fingers become relaxed again. Repeat "clawing" movement 12 times.

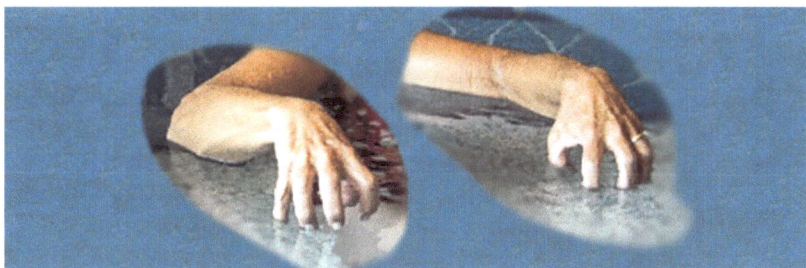

ACTION: This exercise uses the same muscles as the "piano" exercise but emphasizes use of the flexor digitorum brevis and profundus to perform the clawing movement.

Thumb Circles
(The Thumb Does Not Bend)

Helps stretch the thumb tendon and major hand joints near the thumb and increases dexterity and flexibility.

The hands are placed in front of torso, held prone or flat to the water's surface with the palms down.

The thumbs on both hands are rotated inward 12 to 25 thumb rotations.

Then, the thumbs of both hands are rotated outward from for 12 to 25 thumb rotations.

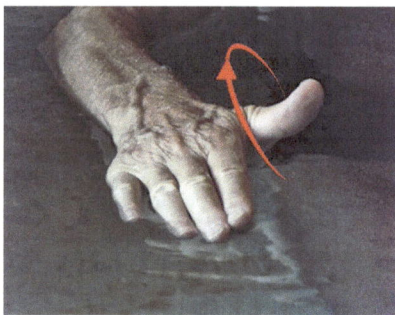

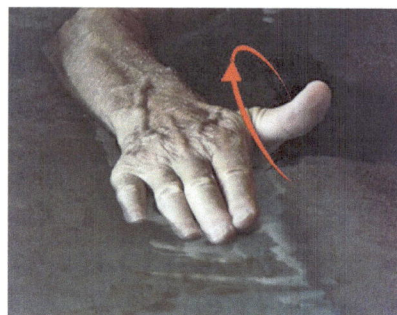

ACTION: In sequence of the muscles being used, the circling motion of the thumbs stretches and contracts the flexor pollicis longus, the abductor pollicis, the extensor pollicis, and the adductor pollicis.

Thumb Stretches

Helps additional thumb movement, stretches the major thumb tendon, strengthens wrists.

The arms and hands are placed in front of the torso, flat palms are floating on the water's surface. The thumbs on both hands are pulled under the palms of the hands and brought back out again. Repeat 12 to 15 times.

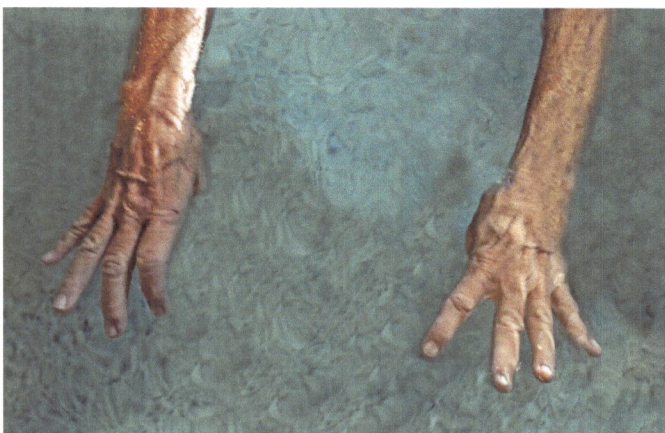

ACTION: Moving the thumb away from the palm is thumb flexion and is performed primarily by the flexor pollicis longus and brevis muscles. Bringing it back in line with the other fingers is thumb extension and is primarily performed by the extensor pollicis longus and brevis muscles.

Wrist Circles

Helps to improve wrist flexibility and dexterity.

Arms and hands are held in front of the torso with the palms down.

Elbows are slightly bent as both wrists circle at the same time, first, inward and then, outward.

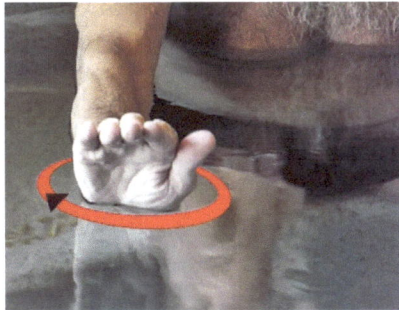

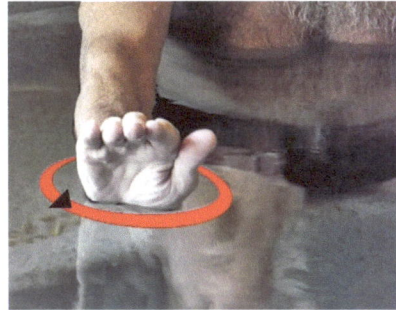

ACTION: Having the palms face down activates the forearm pronators. Moving the wrist down uses the wrist flexors, moving it towards the thumb side of the hand uses the wrist radial deviators, moving it upwards uses the wrist extensors and moving it towards the pinky side of the hand uses the wrist ulnar deviators.

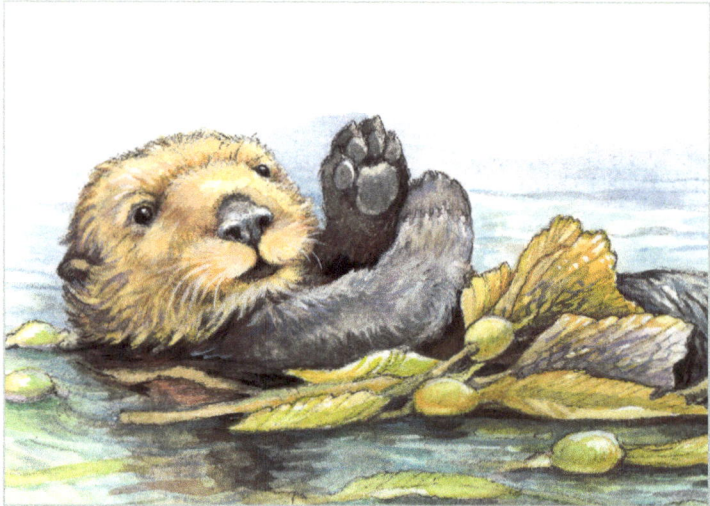

MONDAY

"Marti, I am so indebted to you for your water aerobics instruction. I was in the Air Force and had numerous surgeries including orthoscopy, reconstruction, and hip replacement. During my second hip replacement, my femur was accidentally split. I was in a lot of pain.
I came to my first water aerobics class using a walker and was so very depressed. In less than a month, I was off my walker. I had so much FUN in the class and feel amazing! I am now doing lap swimming. THANK YOU SO VERY MUCH." – Don A.

Monday Pre-Exercise Muscle Information

This section includes cardio exercises. Cardio exercises are important for many reasons. They strengthen the heart, reduce the risk of several diseases, improve lung capacity and naturally boost energy. They are great for mental health, improving the immune system and enhancing sleep.

Cardio exercises can reduce blood pressure and help fight cholesterol. They can also reduce insulin and insulin sensitivity.

Being in the water lets you exercise without putting the full force of gravity on your joints. On land the force on your joints can be six times your body weight. In water, you reduce that force. The water buoyancy cushions the joints to make exercising feel effortless. Moving against the water, the resistance makes muscles work harder. You are toning muscles more effectively than you would on land.

Circulation is increased as the water is always pulsating against the body. You are strengthening muscles around each joint. You also experience less overall pain. Simply changing a direction in the water works a totally different muscle group.

In the jogging exercises, the stability of the two-leg stance is lost; one foot is always elevated off the pool floor. There is a dynamic change in posture. The body is in constant motion shifting from side to side as one leg is lifted from the pool floor and the other is seeking momentary stability on the pool floor. If the torso was not shifting over the leg on the pool floor, the body would fall sideward toward the leg which is not on the pool floor. Walking on a flat surface has the same dynamic of the torso shifting over the leg on the ground as the opposite leg swings forward in preparation to become the stance leg. These exercises are beneficial to walking and balance, such as lifting dishes into and out of cupboards or carrying grocery bags.

Front Kick/Back Kick

Helps balance, coordination, flexibility, strengthens pelvic and lower body muscles.

NOTE: Avoid this exercise if you have had any type of hip replacement.

Begin the exercise with a hop on the left foot. The right knee is swung to the front; the leg straightens and gives two rapid kicks forward using a flat foot. The left arm is thrust forward; the right arm is pulled back to the waist with a bent elbow to maintain better balance and help assist leg extension.

The leg is then swung backwards for two kicks; bending the knee as it passes the torso and straightening the leg with as flat a foot as possible. When the leg is swung to the back, it is not always possible to lift the leg as high in the water as was possible when kicking to the front. This is repeated 25 times or as many times as possible. One movement of front to back is one repetition.

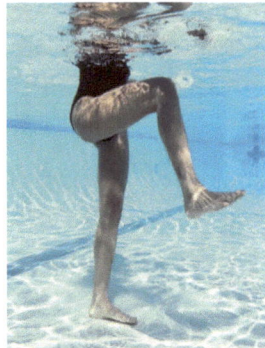

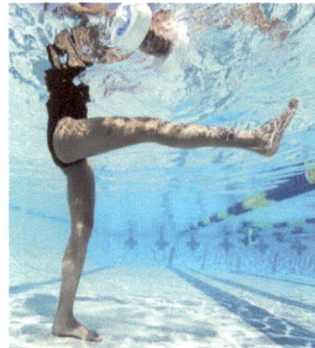

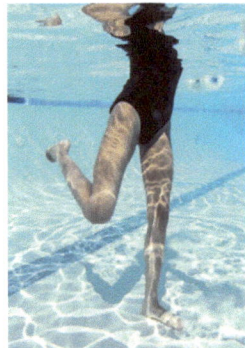

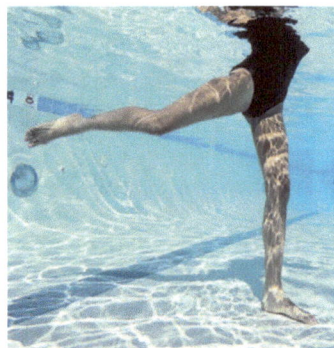

Repeat the exercise 25 more times, changing to execute the above exercise on the left side, two front kicks with a flat foot and two back kicks. Jogging begins after this exercise and before the next exercise.

ACTION: Hopping from one foot to the other involves the hip extensors, knee extensors and ankle plantar flexors to generate force off of the ground. Swinging the leg forward activates the hip flexors while straightening the leg with a flat foot involves the knee extensors and ankle dorsiflexors. Pushing the arm forward uses the shoulder flexors and elbow extensors while pulling the other arm back involves the shoulder extensors and elbow flexors. Swinging the leg back is primarily performed by the hip extensors and knee flexors.

Alternating Side Kicks

Helps balance, stability, and strengthens the ankles, knees, and pelvic muscles.

NOTE: Avoid this exercise if you have any type of hip replacement.

Hold the weights out to the side of the torso. Hop on the left foot kicking the right foot, with a flat foot, out to the side towards the right weight.

Keep holding the weights out to the side of the torso with arms outstretched.

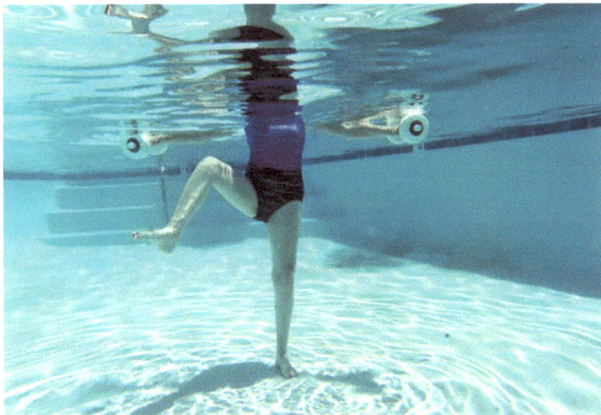

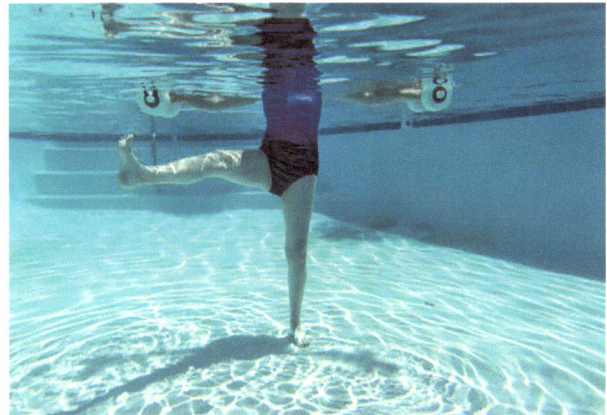

Now, hop on the right foot; then kick to the side towards the right weight with a flat foot to the outstretched arm.

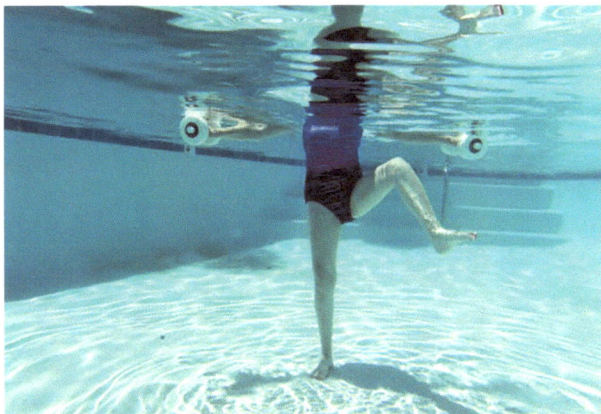

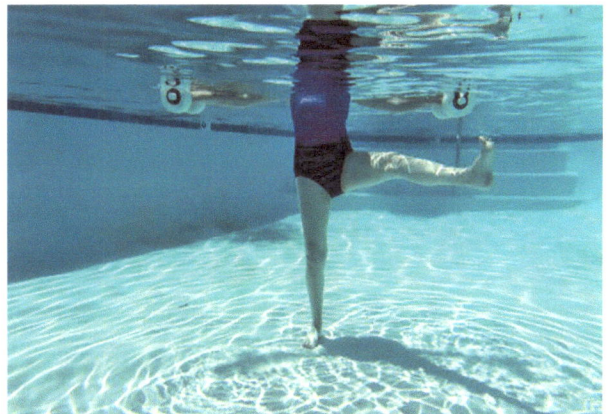

One right kick and one left kick to each side is one repetition. Repeat 25 times.

ACTION: The stance leg requires activation of the hip abductors and extensors to maintain a stable trunk position. The kicking leg strengthens the hip abductors, knee extensors and ankle dorsiflexors. Hopping to the other leg uses the hip extensors, knee extensors and ankle plantar flexors in a rapid contraction to generate force.

"The Core" Exercise

Helps strengthen abdominal muscles, legs, arms, and shoulders.

NOTE: Avoid this exercise if you have had any type of hip replacement.

The legs are stretched out in front of the torso with the weights held out to the side. Knees and ankles are held together as twenty to thirty small kicks are performed with the heels.

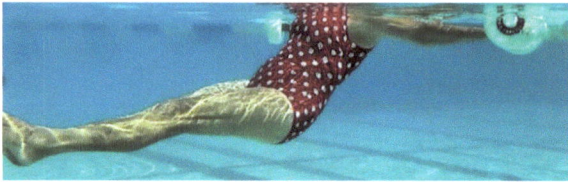
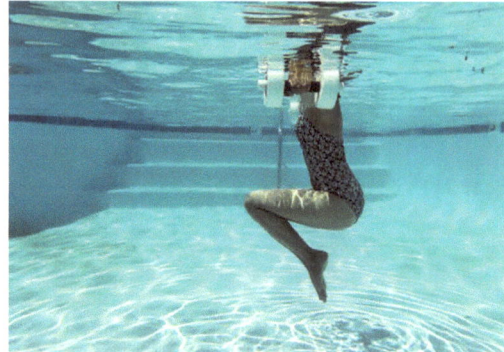

Then, the knees are bent as the torso curls to place the legs to the rear of the torso. The weights are moved and placed together under the chest to keep the torso elevated. The legs, after the curled-up position, are stretched out behind the torso.

ACTION: Holding the arms out to the side and keeping the body floating is activation of the shoulder adductors. The trunk flexors must also be active to stabilize the body position and allow the legs to kick from a stable torso. Kicking utilizes alternating contractions of the hip flexors and extensors with an isometric contraction of the knee extensors and ankle plantar flexors. Curling the knees up towards the chest is primarily targeting the trunk and hip flexors.

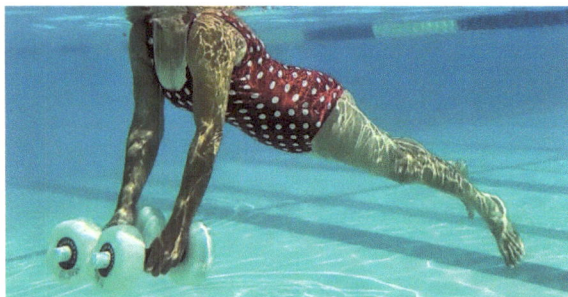
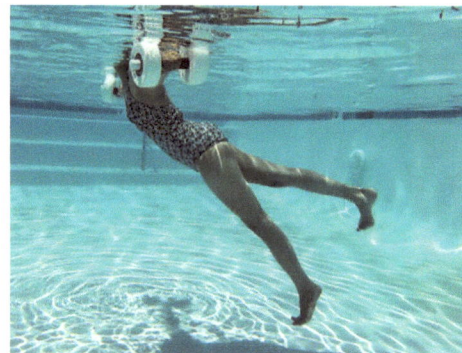

Twenty to thirty small kicks are performed with the toes as the feet are kept flat. The weights are moved back to the outstretched position as the torso is curled again and brought back to the front with the toes up. Repeat the whole process 10 times.

ACTION: Holding the weights under the chest requires a stabilizing contraction of the shoulder flexors, scapular protractors and trunk flexors to maintain a stable torso. Stretching the legs out behind the body utilizes the hip and knee extensors and kicking will involve alternating contractions of the hip flexors and extensors.

Side-to-Side Flutter Kicks

Helps stretch shoulder, back and leg muscles, and improves balance, flexibility, and coordination.

NOTE: Avoid this exercise if you have had any type of hip replacement.

Begin this exercise by jogging. Then, lean gradually to the right, extending the right arm to the right with the weight, arm outstretched. Push the legs to the left. The left arm remains near the torso. Then, begin a series of eight flutter kicks to the left. After the flutter kicks, curl legs to the center of the torso.

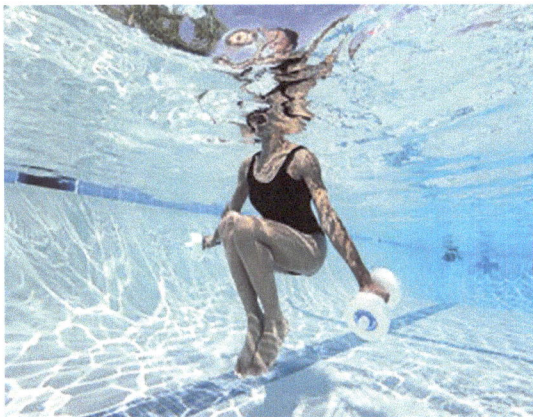
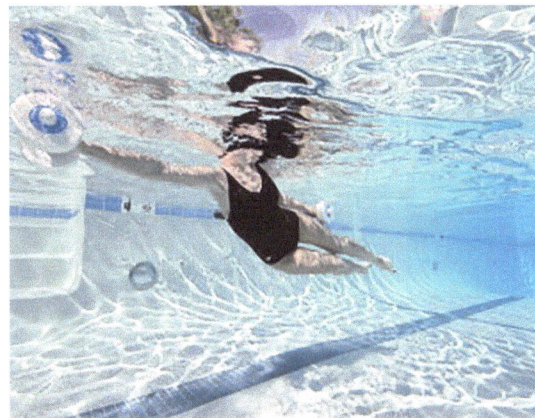

Extend the left arm as the legs uncurl to the left pushing the legs to the right. The right arm remains next to the torso. Begin a series of eight flutter kicks to the right.

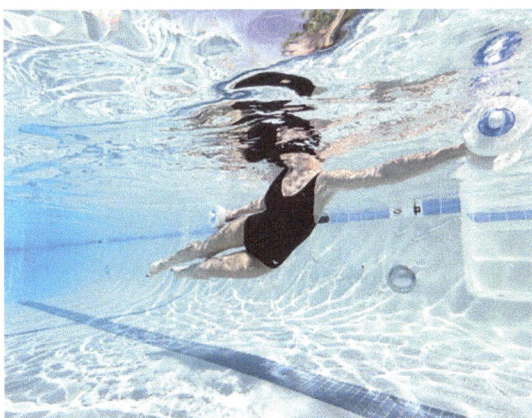

Repeat this whole-body movement 25 times. The legs curl up under the torso as the exercise direction changes. Both arms remain outstretched for balance.

ACTION: With the arm out to the right and the legs flutter kicking to the left, the right shoulder adductors and left trunk side benders are active to maintain this torso position. The flutter kick requires alternating contraction of the hip flexors and extensors. Curling the knees to the chest is a contraction of the trunk flexors.

Double Leg Kicks

Helps strengthen abdominal muscles, hips, and knees.

NOTE: Avoid this exercise if you have had any type of hip replacement.

The arms are held out to the side. Both legs are pulled toward the chest area. Then, both legs are kicked, first to the left.

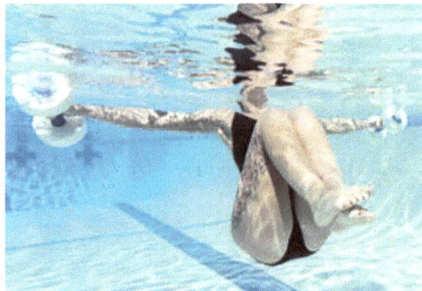

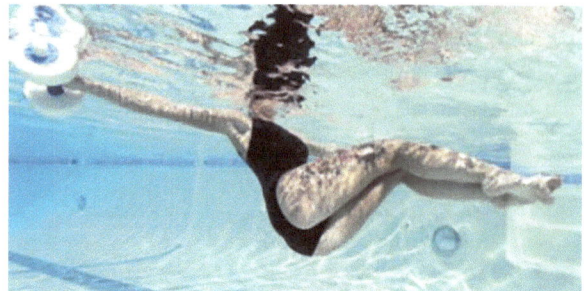

The curled-up legs are pulled back into the chest area and both legs kick to the right.

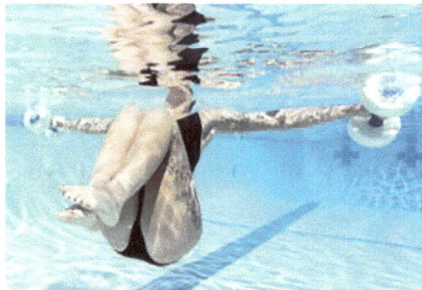

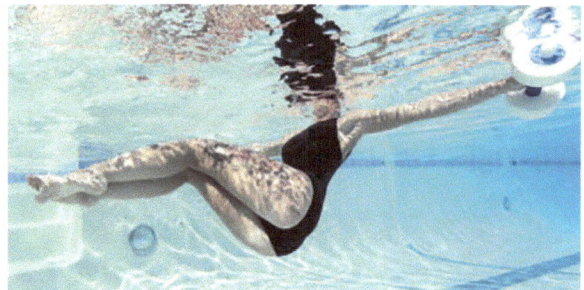

This movement is repeated 25 repetitions, once to the left and then to the right.

ACTION: Holding the arms to the side and keeping the body upright is an isometric contraction of the shoulder adductors and trunk flexors. Pulling the legs towards the chest utilizes the hip flexors and trunk flexors while keeping the legs together requires a contraction of the hip adductors. Kicking the legs to the left utilizes the left trunk rotators, left hip external rotators and right hip internal rotators. Kicking the legs to the right uses the opposite muscles.

Knees to Chest with a Jump

Helps strengthen shoulders, hips, and knees, stabilizing the pelvic area.

The arms are extended out to the side of the torso. In a jumping motion, the knees are pulled toward the chest area. The arms are pulled downward in the water simultaneously.

After curling up, arms and legs are returned quickly to the pool floor as the legs are semi-straightened. Each jumping up, curling inward toward the chest, and returning to the pool floor are counted as one repetition. Repeat for 40 jumps.

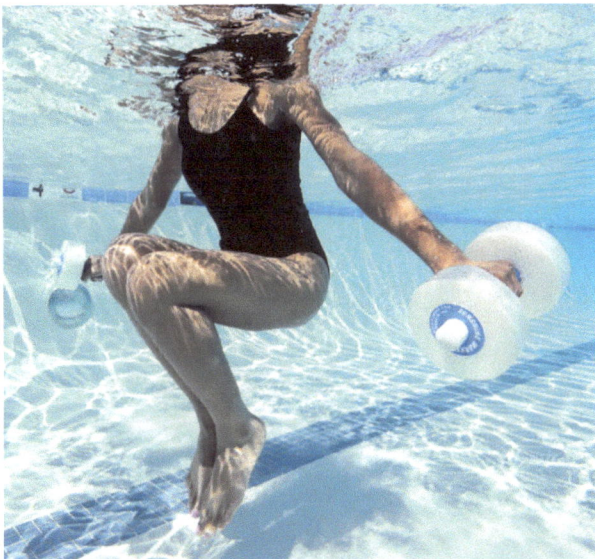

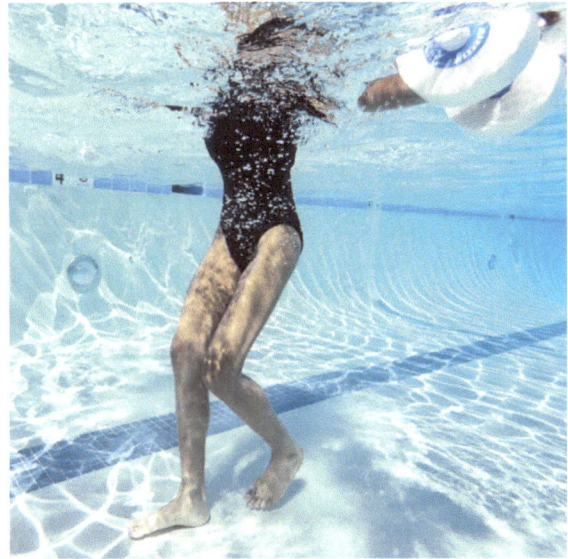

ACTION: Holding the arms to the side of the body and under the water require contraction of the shoulder adductors. Jumping utilizes a quick, concentric contraction of the hip extensors, knee extensors and ankle plantar flexors. Lifting the legs up towards the chest while at the height of the jump requires a quick reversal of the active muscles to engage the hip flexors, knee flexors and ankle dorsiflexors. Extending the legs back down to the floor and landing softly requires an eccentric contraction of mainly the hip and knee extensors.

Three-Way Side Kicks
"The Gretchen"

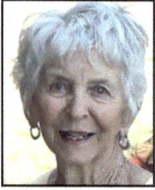

Dedicated to Gretchen Turner, a water aerobics enthusiast.

Helps strengthen and stretch knees, ankles, feet, and lower body muscles. Improves balance and coordination and helps flexibility.

Begin with a hop on the left foot. The right, flat foot kicks to the front, taps the pool as it comes back to the starting position. Then, the right, straight leg, flat foot kicks to the side, taps the pool surface and finally kicks across the torso. This is repeated for 25 repetitions.

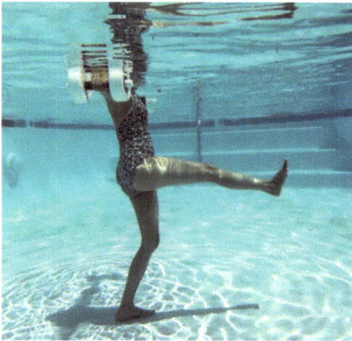

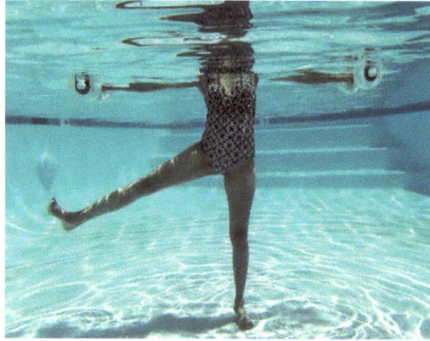

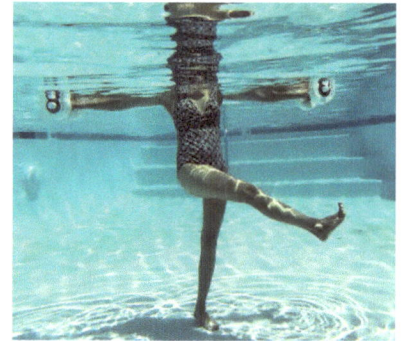

Begin with a hop on the right foot. The left, flat foot kicks to the front, taps the pool as it comes back to the starting position. Then, the left straight leg, flat foot kicks to the side, taps the pool surface and finally kicks across the torso. This is repeated 25 times.

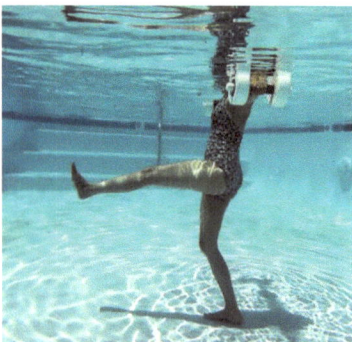

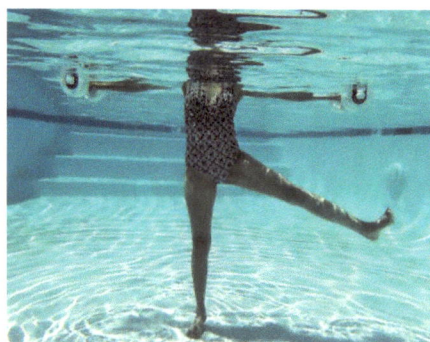

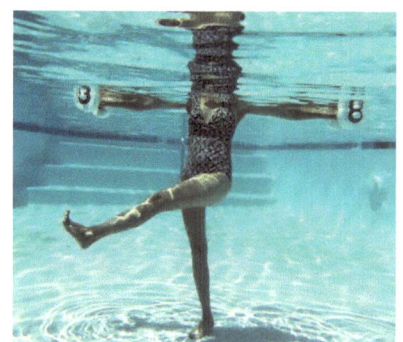

ACTION: To keep the leg straight, a constant contraction of the knee extensors is required. Kicking to the front utilizes the hip flexors, kicking to the side engages the hip abductors and kicking across the body activates the hip adductors.

Forward, Backward, Side-to-Side Running

Helps circulation, cardio, and helps to stabilize the back and pelvic muscles.

The arms are held to the side or on the water's surface. Run forward 8 to 10 steps; backward 8 to 10 steps; and left/right or right/left for 8 to 10 steps.

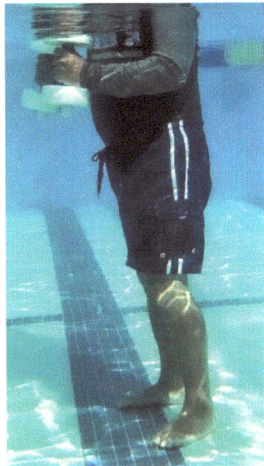

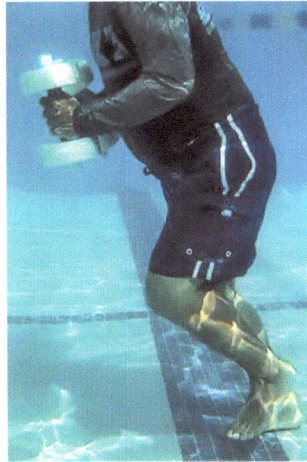

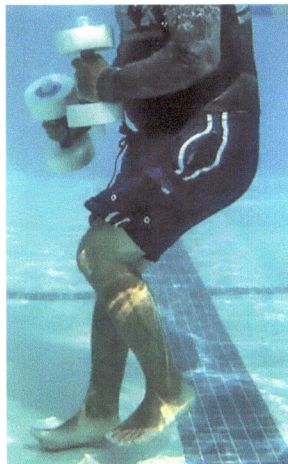

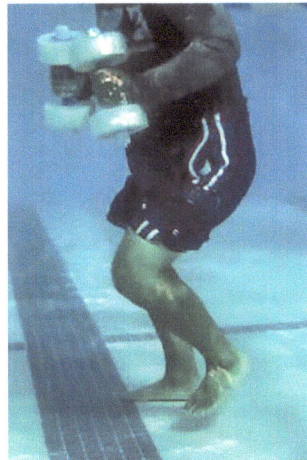

This series of running in a pattern is repeated 4 times.

ACTION: Holding the arms underwater and next to the body in this position engages the shoulder extensors, elbow extensors and wrist ulnar deviators. The running motion engages alternating hip flexors and extensors, knee flexors and extensors and ankle plantar flexors and dorsiflexors. When one leg's flexor is working to lift the leg, the stance leg strengthens the extensors to push into pool floor and support the body. Running forward will further engage the trunk flexors, running backwards will engage the trunk extensors and running to the left/right engages the muscles for trunk side bend.

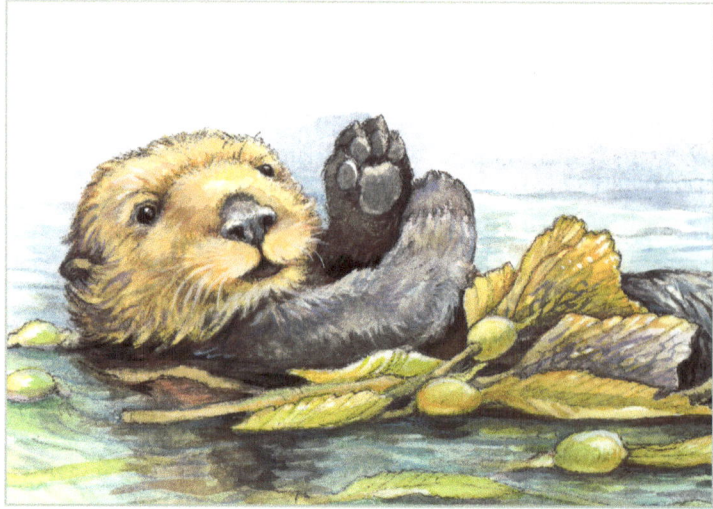

TUESDAY

"*After 16 areas of strokes to my brain and barely alive from a coma, I came to live with a sister who helped me learn to swim again. Then, she enrolled me in Marti's water aerobics class. These whole-body exercises have given me back my strength. I can dive into the deep end of the pool; I can climb out of the pool using the ladder. I no longer consider myself handicapped. Thank you, Marti for helping me become whole again.*" – Donna M.

Tuesday Pre-Exercise Muscle Information

All the exercises in this section which involve the shoulder are using the muscles of the scapula (shoulder blade) to aid the shoulder movement. For any movement to occur in the upper extremity, the shoulder must be held steady to allow controlled movement away (distal) from the shoulder. This dynamic stabilization is made possible by muscles attaching to the shoulder blade. This stabilizing movement of the scapula is essential to the elevation of the arm and is made possible by the coordinated action of the muscles attaching the scapula to the arm, spine, and rib cage.

The scapula is stabilized by the middle and lower trapezius muscles, and the rhomboid muscles. These muscles anchor the scapula and give the arm a stable point from which to generate power. The spine is held erect by the abdominal muscles anteriorly and the spinal muscles posteriorly acting in unison. When the spinal muscles and abdominal muscles contract, they pull on their attachment points on the pelvis, the rib cage and the spine. This double pull gives stability to the torso and the pelvis at the same time.

While performing the shoulder exercises, the chin should remain parallel to the pool bottom. This keeps the chin from rising, and stabilizes the neck. It keeps the neck from arching, or hyperextending, stabilizing the neck. Keeping the chin in this position prevents interference with the stabilizing action of the scapular muscles when there is concurrent shoulder movement.

Foot position for balance and walking:

Normal standing **Semi tandem** **Tandem**

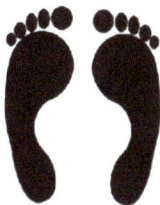 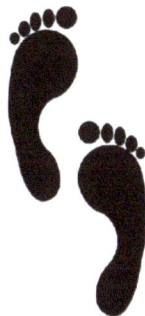 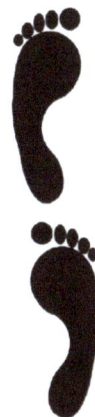

Free Style Arms

Helps improve balance, shoulder, and upper back strength, and increases flexibility.

Stop jogging. A good stationary stance is taken. The right arm reaches out in front holding the weight horizontally. The weight is pulled through the water past the torso to the rear of the torso. As the weight approaches the hip, the forearm internally rotates (pronates), changing the weight orientation from horizontal to vertical and back to horizontal as the right arm rotation is completed.

The left arm begins its rotation when the right arm reaches the hip area. The weight is pulled vertically through the water past the torso to rear of the torso. The wrist rotates to change the direction to that of a horizontal hold on the weight as another arm rotation is completed. Repeat this arm movement 12 to 15 times, alternating the arms.

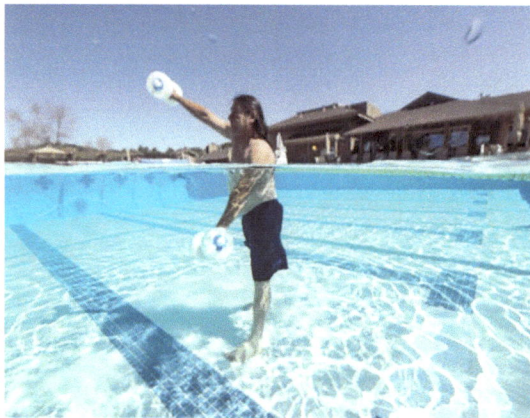

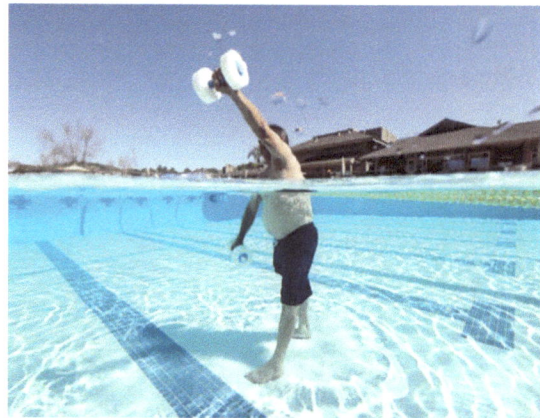

ACTION: Pulling the arm through the water and behind the torso activates the shoulder extensors, elbow extensors and wrist stabilizers. As the arm position changes and passes the hip, the shoulder external rotators and forearm supinators are engaged. Bringing the arm from behind the torso, overhead and back to the front of the body requires activation of the shoulder flexors and isometric activation of the elbow stabilizers.

Back Stroke Arms

Helps posture, range of motion, and balance. Strengthens shoulders and upper body.

Stop jogging. Assume a stationary stance. The left arm pulls the weight vertically forward from the back of the torso and comes out of the water. As the weight held vertically comes toward the head, the arm rotates the weight and holds it horizontally until it reaches the back of the head. The hold on the weight once again becomes a vertical hold as it is pulled through to the front of the torso.

When the right arm reaches the back of the head, the left arm follows through with the same repeated movement.

To experience the maximum body movement, continue this pattern 12 to 15 times.

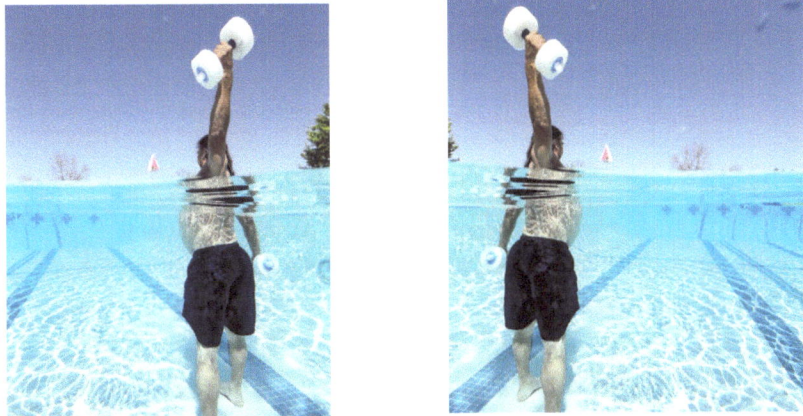

ACTION: Pulling the weight vertically forward from the torso engages the shoulder flexors, elbow flexors and wrist stabilizers. Turning the weight horizontally requires activation of the shoulder internal rotators and forearm pronators as the arm reaches the back of the head. To bring the arm back down engages the opposite muscles: shoulder extensors and external rotators, elbow extensors and forearm supinators.

Alternating Arms

Helps strengthen shoulders, arms and upper body muscles. Stretches upper back and lateral (side) abdominal muscles. Increases range of motion of the arms, improving overall balance.

Maintain a stationary stance with the left foot in front of the torso, facing forward. The right, straight arm is pulled back and forth next to the torso; the left, straight arm is pulled back and forth next to the torso. Both the right, straight arm and the left, straight arm are alternating pushing and pulling next to the torso. Repeat alternating of left/right straight arms 12 times.

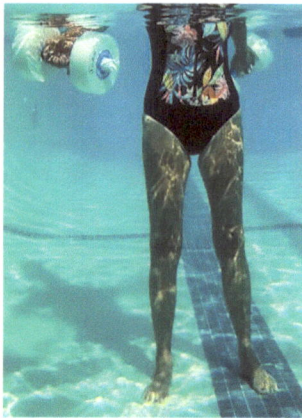

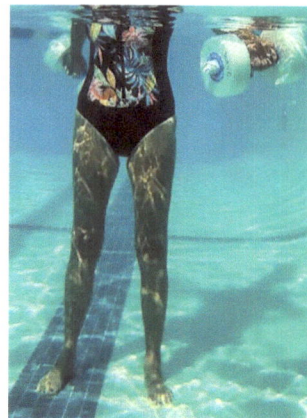

ACTION: Maintaining a straight arm throughout this exercise requires an alternating isometric contraction of the elbow extensors on the way forward and the elbow flexors on the way back. Keeping the palm down throughout the movement requires stabilization by the forearm pronators. Moving the whole arm in front of the torso requires a concentric contraction of the shoulder flexors and moving it behind the torso is a concentric contraction of the shoulder extensors.

Double Arm Pull

Helps strengthen shoulders, arms, wrists, neck, and upper back muscles. Increases body stability throughout the torso.

The torso is facing forward. Feet are firmly placed on the pool floor. Weights are held horizontally on the surface of the water. The straight arms pull both weights to the hips and push them back up.

Repeat this pull/push with straight arms 12 times.

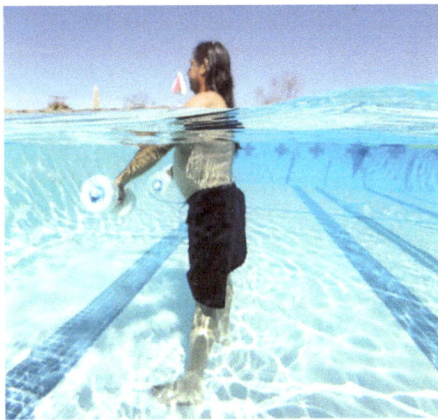

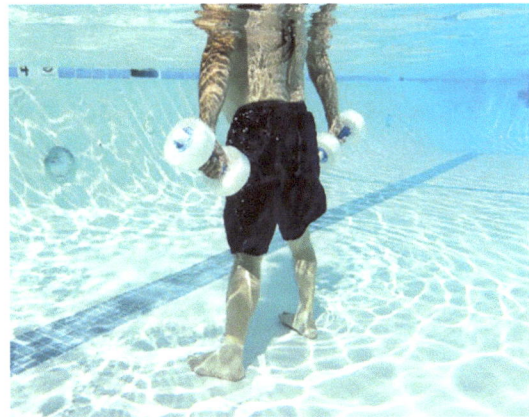

ACTION: Pulling the arms down to the side of the body requires a concentric contraction of the shoulder extensors, and isometric contractions of the forearm pronators and elbow extensors. To maintain a stable torso position, an isometric contraction of the trunk flexors and extensors is required. To allow the arms to come back to the surface slowly requires an eccentric contraction of the same muscles used to pull the weights down to the side.

NOTE: The next 3 exercises are done in succession. All the exercises are first done on the right side; then the same exercises are performed and completed on the left side.

"Sawing Wood"
(Sideways Push/Pull)

Helps balance, range of motion, and strengthens arms, shoulders, knees, and ankles.

Stop jogging.. Assume a good stationary stance. The arms are held out to the side. The left foot is pointed to the left weight; the right arm holds the weight vertically, near the torso. The right arm, which is holding the weight close to the torso, pushes/pulls the weight back and forth near the waist or hip 12 times/pulses.

The stance is reversed. The torso moves toward the right. The right foot is pointed to the right weight, which is moved and held to the right. The left arm holds the weight, vertically, near the waist by the torso, or close to the hip. The left arm pushes/pulls the weight toward the left weight 12 times.

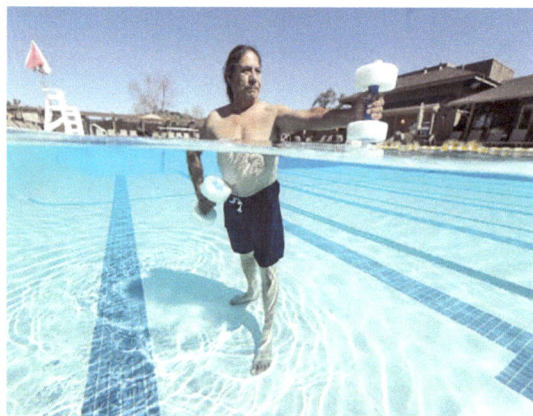

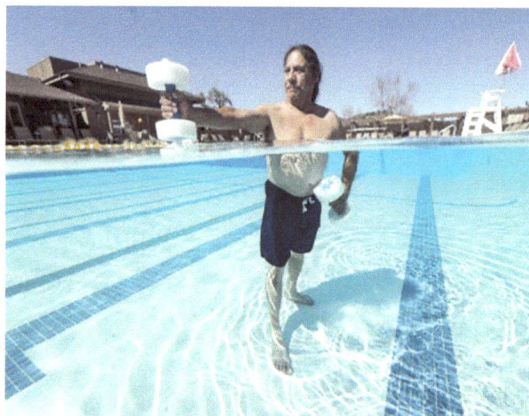

ACTION: The target arm is the one next to the torso performing the forward and back motion. To push the weight forward in the water, there must be contraction of the shoulder flexors, elbow extensors, and forearm stabilizers on both sides of the forearm. Because the weight is underwater, there is also a balancing, eccentric contraction of the shoulder extensors to keep the weight from popping up to the surface of the water.

Side Pushing Arms with a Circular Movement

Helps balance, range of motion, and coordination. Strengthens arms, wrists, and upper torso muscles.

Keep the same position as "the Sawing Wood" exercise (see previous page). The torso remains facing toward the left and the left weight. The right arm is still holding the weight near the waist or hip. The weight is pushed forward, coming to the surface of the water. The arm makes a circular movement away from the torso. Then, the arm completes the circle returning to the torso. This circular movement is repeated for 12 times.

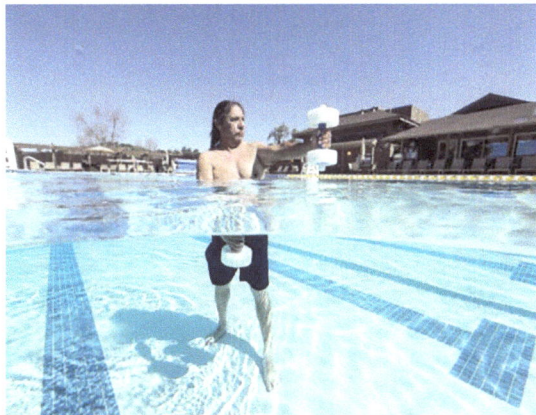

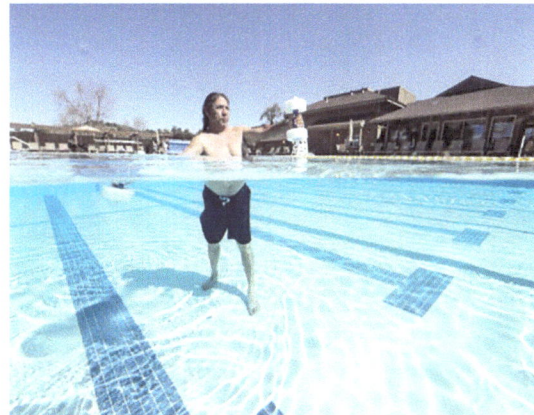

Then the torso faces the right and the right weight. The left arm is still holding the weight near the waist or hip from the previous exercise. The weight is pushed forward, coming to the surface of the water. The left arm makes a circular movement away from the torso. Then, the arm completes the circle returning to the torso. This circular movement is repeated for 12 times.

ACTION: Moving the weight in a clockwise circle across the top of the water requires activation of the following muscle groups in succession: shoulder horizontal abductors, elbow flexors, shoulder horizontal adductors, and elbow extensors (exact muscles listed in the glossary). Keeping the weight underwater requires an isometric contraction of the shoulder extensors, core stabilizers and wrist stabilizers.

Arm Behind Torso, Push/Pull

Helps strengthen elbow, wrist, shoulder, and upper arm muscles.

Right side: A good stance is maintained. The left arm remains outstretched toward the left. The left foot points toward the left weight. The right arm, holding the weight horizontally, is brought down to the hip and then brought back up toward the waist. From the elbow, the right arm is pushed/pulled backward and forward from the waist to extend behind the torso and hip. The weight does not come above the surface of the water. This motion is repeated 6 to 12 times depending upon a person's arm strength.

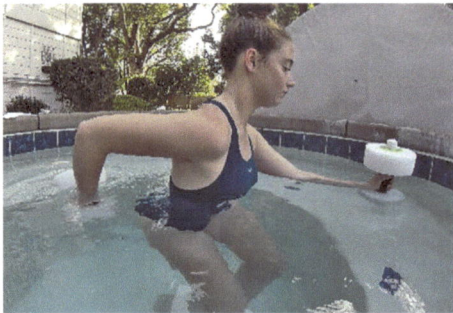
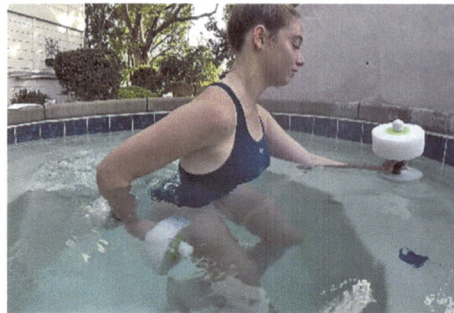

ACTION: Getting the arm to the starting position behind the torso and hip requires activation of the shoulder extensors and maintaining a bent elbow position throughout the exercise requires an isometric, stabilizing contraction of the elbow flexors and extensors. Pushing the arm forward toward the waist strengthens the shoulder flexors. The stance from the previous exercises remains the same and requires a constant contraction of the pelvic and trunk stabilizers to keep the torso stable while the arms move.

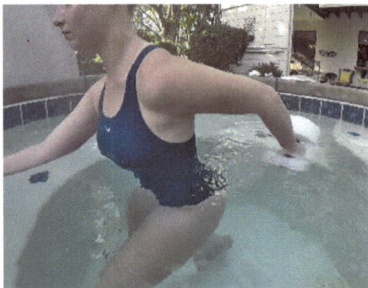
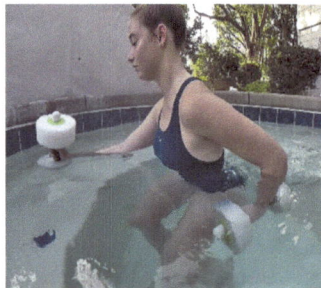
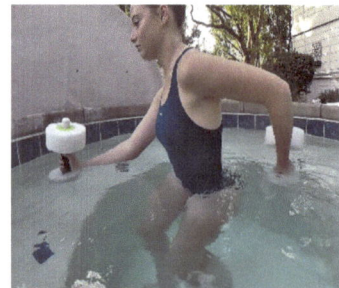

Left side: Repeat this exercise with the left arm as shown in the above photos.

ACTION: This uses the same muscles as previously stated, but on the other side of the body.

Leg Kicks with Boxing Arms

Helps increase endurance, cardio fitness, coordination, and body stability. Strengthen arms, shoulders, and upper back.

The exercise begins by jogging in place. Jog toward the right about 8 to 10 steps. The jogging continues as you kick out in front of the torso, with a flat foot, alternating kicks. Alternate the kicks right and left 15 counts. Jog back to the left and alternate the right/left kicks for 15 counts. Each time, the right and left kicking motion is counted as one kick.

Repeat and add boxing arms to the fast kicking found below.

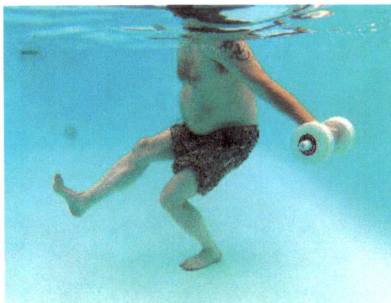

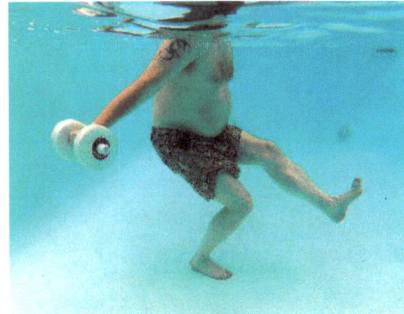

ACTION: Jogging requires alternating contraction of the hip flexors and extensors, knee flexors and extensors and ankle plantar flexors and dorsiflexors. Due to the alternating contractions, the pelvic stabilizers must be active throughout the entire exercise to keep the torso still. Jogging to the right further engages the right hip abductors and left hip adductors. Kicking out in front of the body with a flat foot engages the knee extensors and ankle dorsiflexors. Bringing the foot back to the ground activates the knee flexors and ankle plantar flexors. Jogging back to the left engages the left hip abductors and right hip adductors.

The person then jogs and punches 15 times in front of the torso, alternating the arm punches with a crossover of the opposite arm. At the conclusion of the punching, the person jogs back and to the left about 8 to 10 jogs/steps.

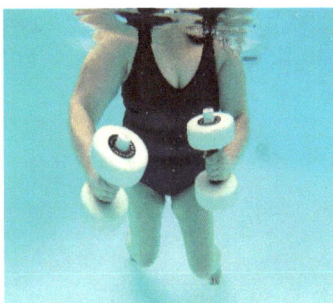

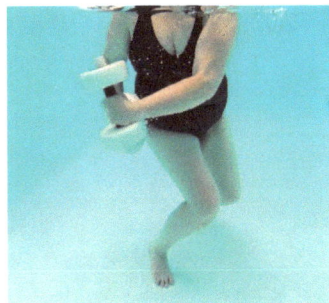

Repeat the exercise, jogging to the left side this time as in the fast-kicking exercise continuing with the same pattern.

ACTION: This exercise uses the same muscles as the jogging but with the addition of activation of the shoulder flexors and elbow extensors when punching forward and utilization of the shoulder extensors and elbow flexors when pulling the arm back to the side. To keep the torso stable, an isometric contraction of the pelvic and trunk stabilizers is required.

47

Hopping on One Foot with a Straight Leg/Kick
(The straight leg kick is to the front of the torso; then, to the side of the torso)

Helps improve balance, foot, knee and hip strength.

During this exercise, the weights are held out to the side with straight or slightly bent arms to help balance. The right leg is held straight out in front with toes pointing upward. Hop on the straight left leg using the ball of the foot for 40 hops. Then do 40 kicks toward the weight. Jog 25 times in between the hopping repetitions.

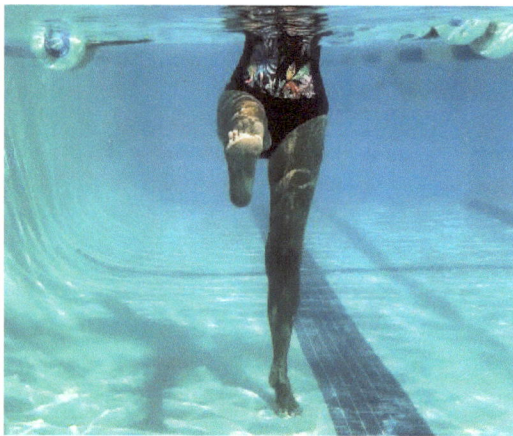

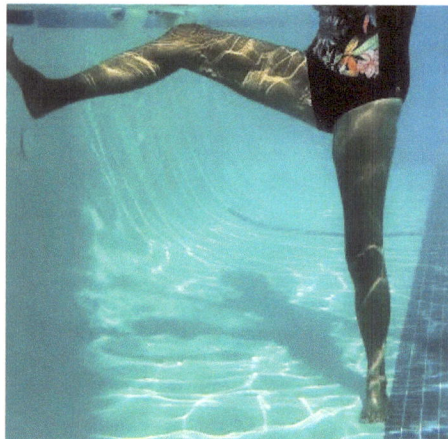

Repeat this exercise with the left leg.

ACTION: Obtaining the single leg stance position and lifting the right leg involves activation of the left hip and knee extensors and ankle stabilizers. On the right leg, the hip flexors, knee extensors and ankle dorisflexors are active. Keeping the torso upright and stable involves activation of the trunk stabilizers. Hopping on the left leg on the ball of the foot mainly targets the ankle plantar flexors and kicking out towards the weight targets the knee extensors.

Brake 'n Clutch Kicking

Helps improve agility, coordination, knees hips and lower body stability

The right foot, held flat, kicks rapidly to the front of the torso (like putting the brake on a car) 8 times.

The left foot, held flat, kicks rapidly to the front (like pushing a clutch on a stick shift car) 8 times.

This brake-and clutch movement is repeated twice with each leg before jogging resumes.

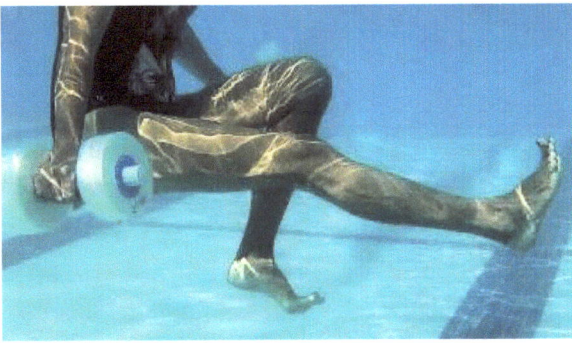

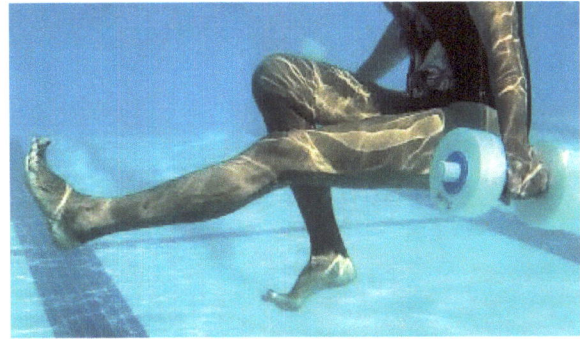

NOTE: Some people feel more comfortable leaning the torso slightly back at the shoulders.

ACTION: Maintaining this floating position in the water requires activation of the shoulder extensors, elbow extensors and wrist stabilizers. The trunk and pelvic stabilizers must also be active to keep the torso still while the legs move. Holding the foot flat engages the ankle dorsiflexors in an isometric contraction to keep it in this position throughout the exercise. Kicking the foot out straight requires activation of the knee extensors and bringing it back towards the body will engage the knee flexors.

"Football" Running

Helps strengthen lower legs, improves accuracy of foot movement, and helps cardio fitness.

Run to the right or left using the ball of the foot with tiny steps for 8 to 10 small running steps. Then run in place rapidly for 30 seconds. Reverse directions and run in place rapidly for 30 seconds. Repeat (like running with steps through the center of a tire) 3 or 4 times.

Run to the right or left on the ball of the foot with tiny steps 8 to 10 times. Then, run in place rapidly for 30 seconds.

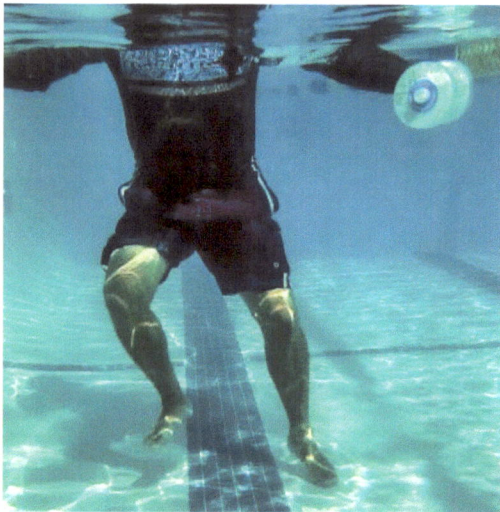

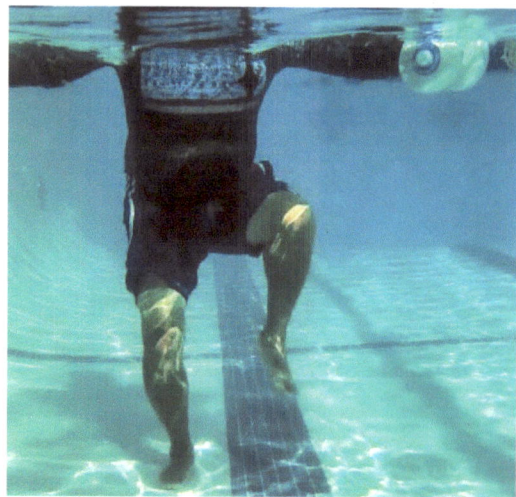

ACTION: Running requires alternating activation of the hip flexors and extensors, knee flexors and extensors and ankle plantar flexors and dorsiflexors. To maintain trunk and pelvic position, the trunk and pelvic stabilizers are constantly active in an isometric contraction to keep the body from swaying back and forth. Running to the right involves additional activation of the right hip abductors and left hip adductors. To perform a forceful acceleration forward, this requires a quick, concentric contraction of the hip extensors, knee extensors and ankle plantar flexors of the leg that touches the ground. Forcefully accelerating backwards requires contraction of mainly the knee extensors on the leg that touches the ground.

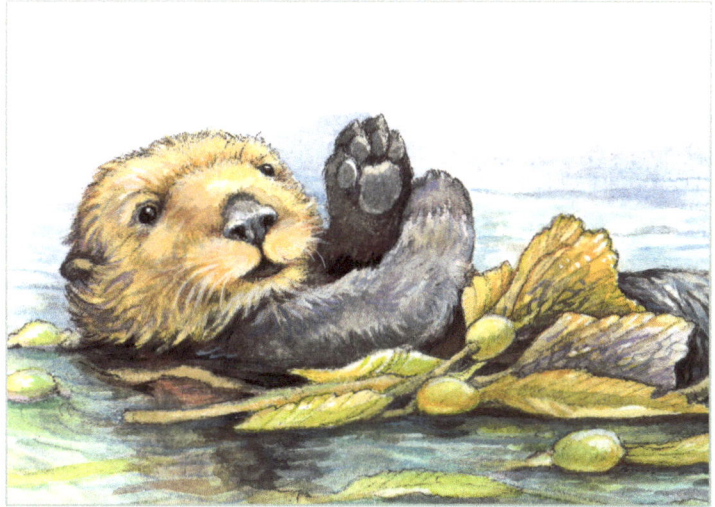

WEDNESDAY

"After a fall from hiking, I had to use a walker to get around the house. The following day, limping, I attended a water aerobics class. The leg exercises and lots of water movement were a great help. I was able to give up the walker that evening. By the next day, I was able to walk without a limp. Water aerobics has become my favorite class." – Linda C.

Wednesday Pre-Exercise Muscle Information

NOTE: Many of the exercises within this section are NOT recommended for people who have had back surgery or total hip replacement.

In shallow water, lean back on your noodle with weights held out to the side and palms up, arms slightly bent. The toes are brought up to the water's surface with the knees and ankles straight and together in front of the torso. It is recommended that a light pressure be exerted by pressing the torso against the noodle. The main function of the noodle is to provide elevation of the arms and shoulders in the water.

In many of these exercises, the arms and legs will be moving simultaneously. Therefore, it is essential that the torso remain erect and stable. The arms and legs are moving at the same time leaving the torso without an anchor point for external stability. By maintaining an erect posture, the torso becomes the anchor for both the legs and arms. Since the body is floating without an anchor, it can only maintain an erect posture for a few moments.

The noodle provides stability for the torso and shoulders in the semi-reclined body position, allowing abdominals and spinal muscles to stabilize the pelvis. With the pelvis stabilized, the muscles attached to the pelvis (proximal attachment) and the thigh (distal attachment) can perform strong contractions.

Stabilizing the torso while moving the lower extremities involves the "core" stabilizers: the transverse abdominis, and multifidi muscles, which are reinforced by the superficial abdominal muscles.

Elevating the torso is a function of the latissimus dorsi assisted by the resistance of the water's buoyancy; pressure downward on the noodle is also a function of the latissimus dorsi.

Side-to-Side Scissor Kick

Helps coordination, pelvic stability. Strengthens legs, and stretches lower back.

NOTE: Avoid this exercise if you have had any type of hip replacement.

With straight legs and foot pointed outward, scissor the legs from side to side. The scissor strokes are very short- approximately shoulder distance apart. The right leg moves across the left leg; the left leg moves across the right leg alternating the legs. Repeat 25 times.

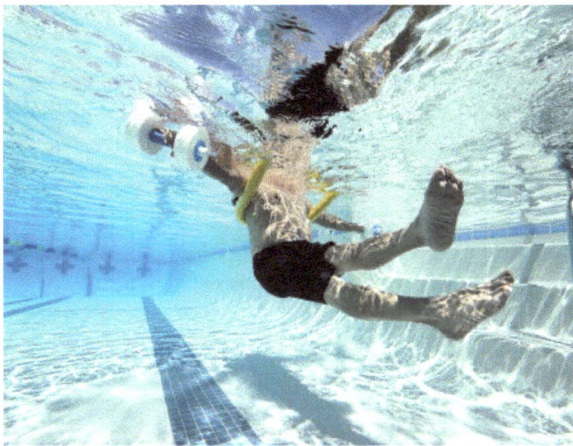

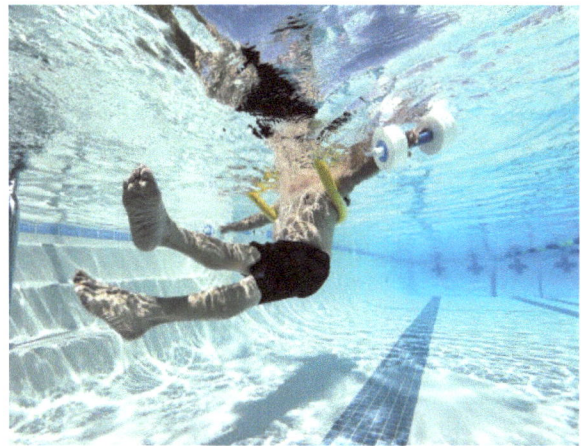

ACTION: Holding the arms out to the side to support the body in a floating position requires an isometric contraction of the shoulder adductors while holding the legs out in front of the body is an isometric contraction of the hip flexors and trunk stabilizers. Moving both legs to the side requires activation of the hip abductors and bringing them back together and over the other is mainly an action of the hip adductors. It is important to perform a tightening action of the abdominal muscle as well as to maintain pelvic stability and avoid rolling over to the side.

Mini-Crunches
(This exercise is assisted by water buoyancy)

Helps strengthen and stretch abdominal muscles. Strengthens arms and shoulders. Increases range of motion of upper legs and knees

The right ankle is placed above the left knee, making the number 4 shape with the right leg. The right knee/leg is then pulled toward the right armpit/shoulder. Then, it is pushed back to the starting position. When the knee is brought up to the armpit/shoulder a better pulling movement can be executed if the weights are brought forward toward the stationary leg. The back/forth movement is repeated 25 times with the right knee/leg.

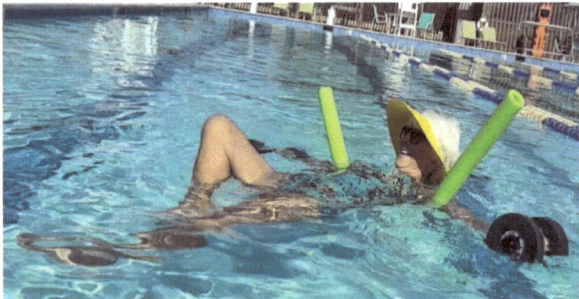

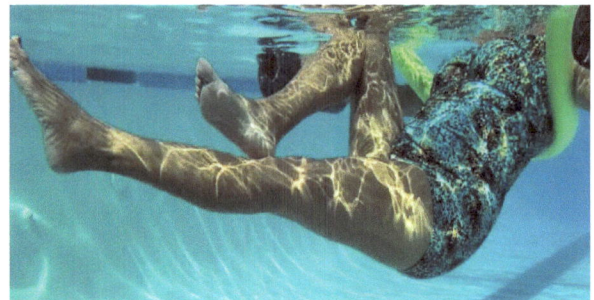

Repeat the entire movement, starting with the left ankle.

ACTION: Bringing the leg into the figure 4 shape is the primary action of the Sartorius muscle located on the inside aspect of the leg. This also activates the other hip flexors, knee flexors and hip external rotators. Pulling the knee/leg towards the shoulder is completed by the hip flexors, knee flexors and trunk flexors. The hip extensors, knee extensors and trunk stabilizers are activated to avoid arching the torso in the water while pushing the legs back to the starting position. Throughout the exercise, the shoulder adductors and extensors are active in an isometric, stabilizing contraction to keep the body afloat. The elbow extensors and wrist extensors engage especially when the straight arms are bought forward.

Water Pilates

Helps strengthen arms, shoulders, upper and lower back, and abdominal muscles.

Lean back on the noodle with weights held straight out to the side. The noodle becomes like a horseshoe behind the shoulders. The toes are brought up and raised to the water's surface, the knees and ankles are held together. The weights are then moved next to the thighs and held there.

With one big pull-down movement of the weights, the heels of the feet become elevated. The arms are kept straight and next to the torso.

The weights are pulsated, a small down/up movement next to the hips, for approximately 40 pulses. Rest for approximately 30 seconds before beginning another big pull-down movement.

This exercise can be done for as many big pull-down movements as a person can manage. The pulses are always the same, 40 pulses for each pull-down. It is recommended that you repeat this exercise at least ten times.

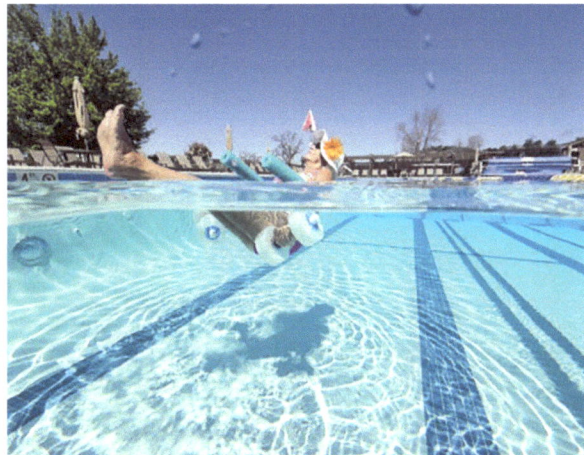

ACTION: Leaning back into the noodle allows the buoyancy of the water to keep the body afloat, but the trunk stabilizers are still required to perform an isometric contraction to keep the body from moving around. Raising the toes to the surface of the water is a contraction of the hip flexors, knee extensors, ankle dorsiflexors and trunk flexors. Holding the legs together will strengthen the hip adductors. Bringing the arms next to the hips requires a strong, concentric contraction of the shoulder extensors, elbow extensors and wrist stabilizers. Pulsating the arms next to the hips requires alternating concentric to eccentric contractions of the muscle groups listed previously. When the arms are pushed down and the legs come up, this also engages the trunk flexors.

The Chair

Helps improves balance and coordination.　Strengthens lateral (side) abdominals. Improves pelvic stability.

The legs are held out straight in front of the torso.　Lower the legs, bend the knees, and pull them under the torso. The knees are facing forward in sitting position. Keep the back straight and in line with the head. The bent knees are rotated from left to right for 20 to 25 rotations; one left/ right is a rotation.

Then the legs are brought back to the surface and extended in front of the torso for the next exercise.

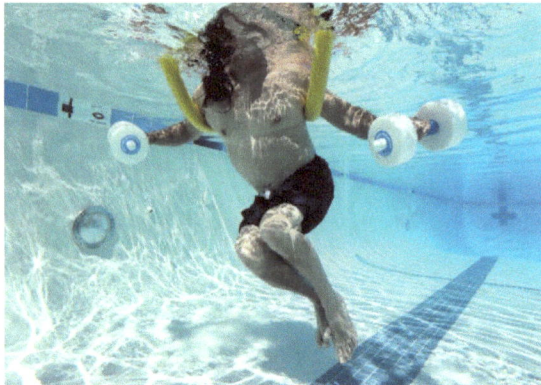

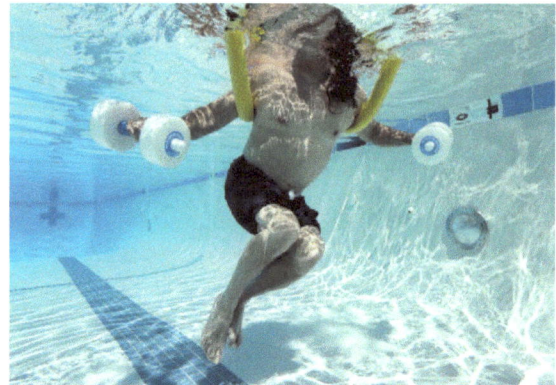

ACTION: Lowering the legs into the starting position of the chair requires contraction of the back extensors, hip extensors and knee flexors. Keeping the legs together and the body still requires isometric contractions of the hip adductors and trunk and pelvic stabilizers. When rotating to the left, the left internal obliques and right external obliques are activated. While rotating to the right, the right internal obliques and left external obliques are activated. Because of the nature of this twisting motion and the action of the muscles required to perform this movement, both sides of the torso are active throughout the entire exercise. Bringing the legs back to the surface of the water and extending them out in front of the body requires contraction of the trunk flexors, hip flexors and knee extensors. The shoulder adductors, elbow and wrist stabilizers are also constantly active to keep the body floating and maintain grip of the weights.

Horizontal Brake/Clutch Movement
(An alternating push/pull movement similar to fast kicking)

Helps knee and hip flexibility. Strengthens lower body and pelvic muscles. Improves arm and shoulder strength.

With the left leg straight and as close to the water surface as possible, lower the right leg about 6 inches below the water's surface. With a flat foot, the right leg is moved about 12 inches, back/forth rapidly approximately 15 times, then both legs are returned to the water's surface.

Keep the right leg straight and as close to the water surface as possible. Lower the left leg about 6 inches below the water's surface. With a flat foot, the left leg is moved about 12 inches, back and forth rapidly about 15 times. This left and right leg sequence is repeated twice or more before completing the exercise.

To finish this exercise, both legs, with ankles together, are lowered about 6 inches under the water's surface to perform the same rapid pull/push movement 15 times.

The legs stay in line with the shoulders and hips throughout this exercise.

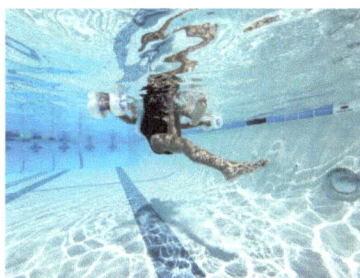

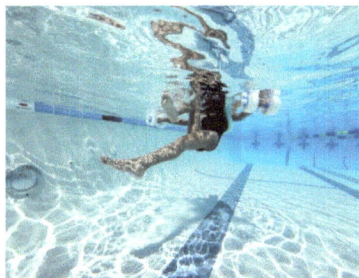

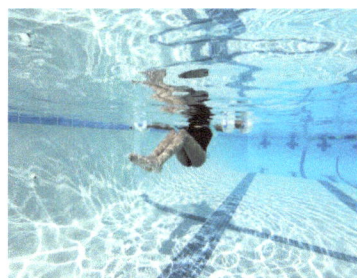

ACTION: Obtaining the starting position along the surface of the water and foot flat is mostly performed by the trunk and pelvic stabilizers with assistance from the water buoyancy. Moving one leg 6 inches beneath the surface of the water with a flat foot engages the hip extensors, knee extensors and ankle dorsiflexors. Moving the leg back and forth in the brake/clutch movement is primarily an alternating contraction of the knee extensors and flexors with a constant contraction of the ankle dorsiflexors. As both legs pull/push, greater exertion on the muscles involved in the single leg motion is achieved. With both legs moving, the transverse abdominus and the core stabilizers are working more intensely.

Leg Pull/Push

Helps coordination and range of motion with the lower torso. Strengthens hip, pelvic and lower back muscles. Strengthen shoulders, arms, upper back and neck.

Lean back on the noodle as it supports the chest and upper torso. Arms are extended to the side holding weights. The legs are extended in front with the toes up. The left leg stays at the water's surface while the right straight leg pulls down and pushes back up to the water's surface. The arms with weights move backward as the leg comes down, and forward as the leg returns to the water's surface. Repeat the right leg movement 25 times

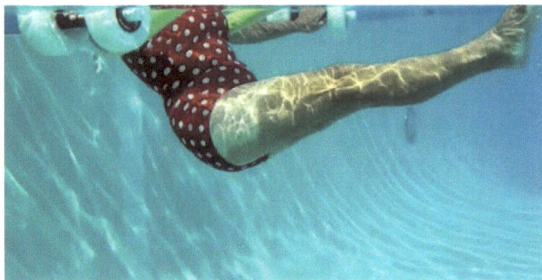

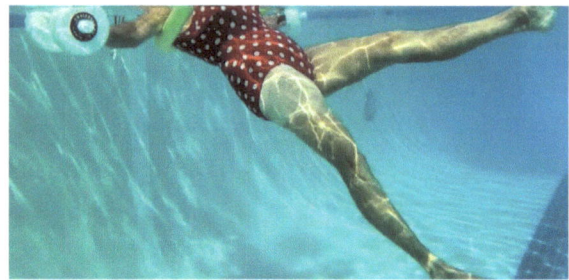

Change legs, keeping the right leg at the water's surface. Pull the left straight leg down and push it back up to the water's surface. Repeat the left leg movement 25 times.

ACTION: Leaning back on the noodle allows for the water buoyancy to assist the trunk stabilizers, keeping the body afloat. Holding the weights out to the side of the body engages the shoulder extensors and adductors in an isometric, stabilizing contraction. Bringing the legs to the surface with toes up engages the hip flexors, knee extensors and ankle dorsiflexors. Bringing one of the legs down primarily activates the hip extensors but also requires constant contraction of the knee extensors and ankle dorsiflexors. Bringing that leg back to the surface primarily strengthens the hip flexors. Stabilizing the torso while moving the lower extremities involves the "core" stabilizers: Transverse Abdominus muscle and Multifidi muscles, which are reinforced by the abdominal muscles.

Ankle Claps

Helps use water pressure to press against inner thighs, increases small muscle movement of the legs. Increases pelvic stability.

Lean back on their noodle with weights held out to the side. The toes are brought up to the water's surface. The knees and ankles are held together. The legs are held straight and out in front of the torso. The toes are lowered about 4-6 inches below the water's surface. Then, the straight legs are moved side to side which pushes the water between the ankles. The ankles should move no further apart than the shoulders. This clapping continues for approximately 100 ankle claps. (This movement is like clapping at a performance.)

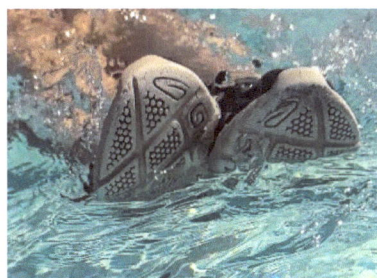

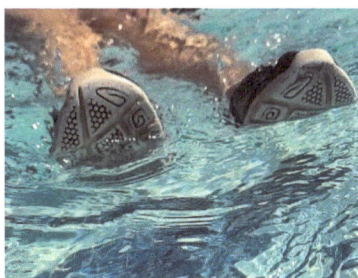

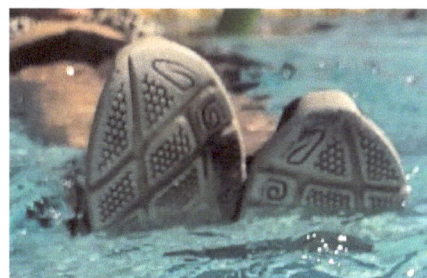

ACTION: Bringing the toes up to the surface of the water requires activation of the hip flexors, knee extensors, ankle dorsiflexors and trunk stabilizers to keep the torso at the surface of the water. Lowering the legs underwater is primarily a contraction of the hip extensors with constant activation of the knee extensors and ankle dorsiflexors. Performing the clapping motion requires alternating activation of the hip abductors (to bring the legs apart) and the hip adductors (to bring the legs back together). To keep the toes pointed up the entire time, the ankle stabilizers must be active to avoid letting the feet move from side to side.

Water Angels

Helps relax the torso, stretches upper back, shoulder and lateral (side) abdominal muscles. Increases pelvic and lower back flexibility. Water buoyancy pulsates the legs improving circulation.

The person leans back on their noodle. The arms with the weights are held near the torso. The legs are straight and held as close to the water's surface as possible.

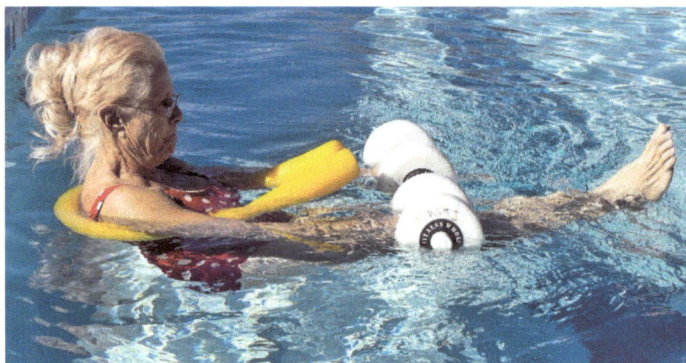

Both the arms and legs are moved at the same time out to the side of the torso and back. This movement is likened to snow angels. The movement is repeated 25 times.

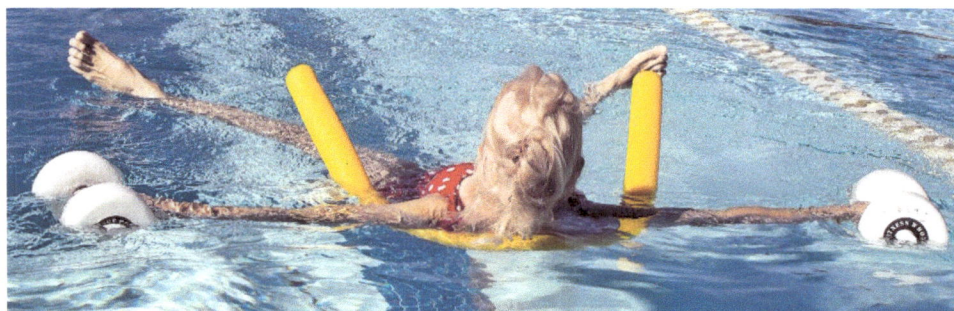

ACTION: The noodle is providing stability for the torso and shoulders in the semi-reclined body position, allowing the abdominals and spinal muscles to stabilize the pelvis. With the pelvis stabilized, the muscles of the lower and upper extremities can perform strong contractions. Bringing the legs out to the side and back together is an alternating contraction of the hip abductors and hip adductors, while bringing the arms out to the side and back together is an alternating contraction of the shoulder abductors and shoulder adductors.

Downward Bent Leg Pull
(The start position with the number 4 bent knee is like the position for mini-crunches)

Helps stretch lower back and thigh muscles. Increases range of hip motion and flexibility. Strengthens lower abdominal muscles.

The right ankle is placed above the left knee, making a number 4 shape with the right leg. Keep the right foot firmly placed on the left knee. The right knee is pulled downward toward the bottom of the pool and pulled back to the starting position. This down/up movement is repeated 15 times before the position is changed.

The left ankle is placed above the left knee, making a number 4 shape with the left leg. Keep the left foot firmly placed on the right knee. The left knee is pulled downward toward the bottom of the pool and pulled back to the starting position. This down/up movement is repeated 15 times.

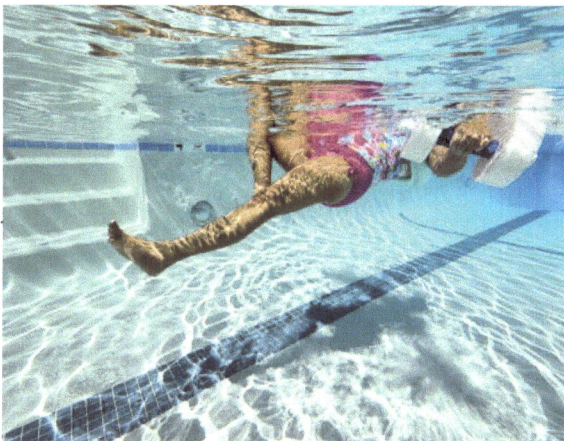

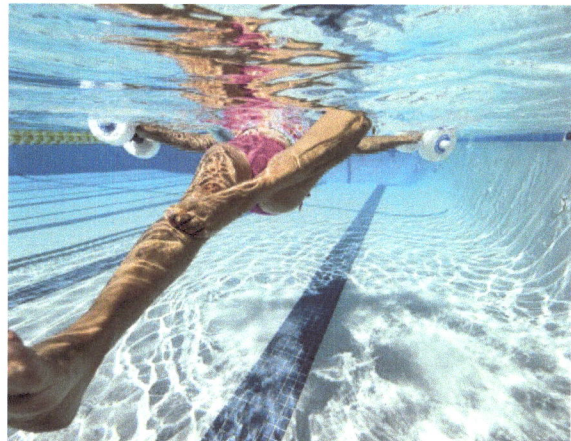

ACTION: Bringing the leg into the figure 4 position as with the mini crunches is the main action of the Sartorius muscle but also engages the other hip flexors, knee flexors and hip external rotators. These muscle groups will have to maintain a strong isometric contraction to keep this figure four position throughout the exercise. Moving the knee down towards the bottom of the pool is hip external rotation and bringing it back to midline is hip internal rotation. These are the muscle groups primarily responsible for the movement of the bent leg. To stabilize the straight leg and the rest of the torso, the trunk and pelvic stabilizers must be constantly active to avoid rolling the entire body from side to side.

Across the Torso, Bent Leg Pull

NOTE: NOT recommended for people who have had back surgery or a total hip replacement.

Helps stretch lower back and pelvic muscles. Stretches and strengthens lower abdominal muscles. Improves range of hip motion and flexibility.

The right ankle is placed above the left knee, making a number 4 shape with the right leg. The right knee is pulled across the torso to the water's surface on the left side and brought back to the starting position. This causes a slight torso roll. The motion across the torso is repeated 15 times before the position is changed.

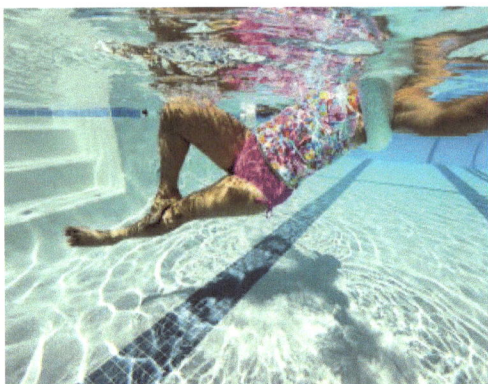

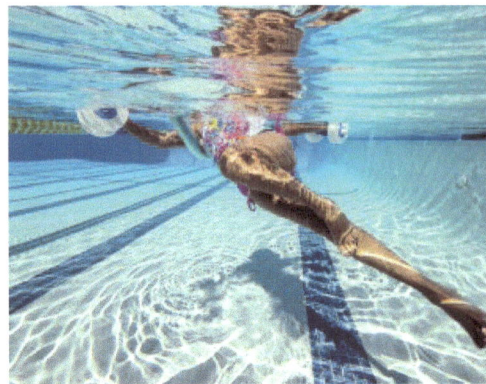

Repeat the exercise, starting with the left ankle placed above the left knee, making a number 4 shape with the left leg. Repeat 15 times.

ACTION: As with the previous exercise, obtaining the figure 4 position requires activation of the Sartorius muscle as well as the hip flexors, knee flexors and hip external rotators. Keeping the opposite leg extended requires constant contraction of the hip extensors and knee extensors throughout the 15 repetitions. As opposed to the previous exercise where the trunk is held still, this exercise requires a trunk and pelvic rotation to obtain the cross-body movement. Pulling the right knee across the torso requires activation of the right internal obliques and left external obliques along with the core stabilizers. Because there is active movement of the trunk in this exercise, the obliques are performing a concentric, forceful contraction as opposed to the last exercise where they were required to perform a stabilizing, isometric contraction to keep the body still.

Wax On and Wax Off

Helps pelvic and spinal flexibility. Strengthens spinal movements in the lower back and torso.

The legs are extended in front of the torso with the toes pointing upward and slightly above the surface of the water. The legs remain on the surface of the water throughout this exercise.

The ankles are held together as the toes are first rotated to the right and then to the left.

This exercise is complete when you have rotated the toes 20 to 25 times, once to the left and once to the right. The legs remain on the water's surface for this exercise.

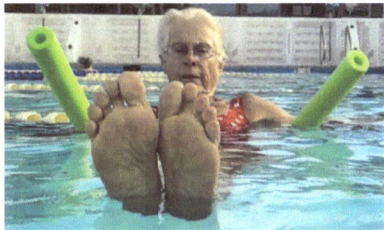

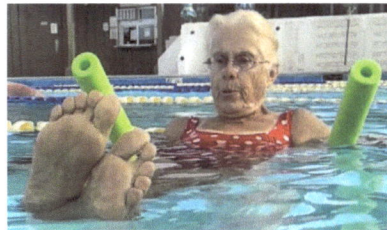

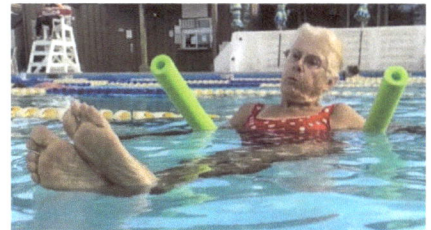

ACTION: Keeping the body along the surface of the water requires contraction of the trunk and pelvic stabilizers. Because this exercise primarily strengthens the hip internal and external rotators, the trunk stabilizers must maintain a strong contraction to avoid letting the trunk roll from side to side. This contraction may involve a conscious squeezing of the abdominals to keep the torso still. Keeping the legs together and toes pointing up activates the hip adductors and ankle dorsiflexors throughout the entire exercise. Rotating the toes to the right activates the right hip external rotators and left hip internal rotators. Rotating the toes to the left activates the left hip external rotators and right hip internal rotators. Regardless of which way the toes are facing, both hips are active throughout the entire exercise.

The Bell

Helps coordination. Increases flexibility of back muscles and hips. Strengthens abdominal muscles and shoulders. Improves body alignment and posture.

This exercise begins with the legs, and ankles held straight together in front of the torso.

The knees are bent with the ankles remaining together. The bent knees are pulled forward to the water's surface; then, the knees are pulled behind the torso.

The forward motion with the knees followed by backward behind the torso, a swinging motion, continues for 12-15 times.

Then the legs are stretched out in front at the completion of the exercise.

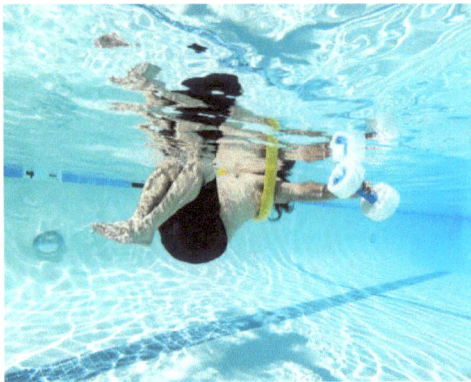

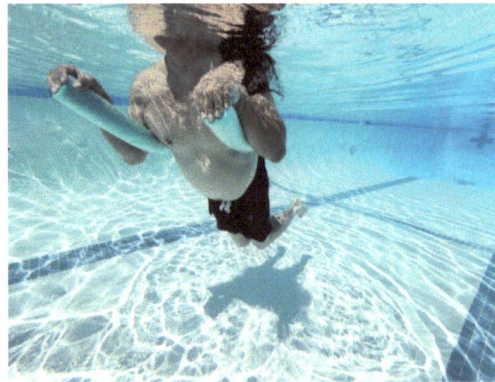

ACTION: This is a full body exercise that requires constant stabilization of the trunk, pelvis and shoulders. The starting position of this exercise with the legs out in front of the body and the torso along the surface of the water requires isometric contractions of the trunk and pelvic stabilizers, hip adductors and shoulder horizontal abductors. Pulling the knees into the chest primarily targets the trunk flexors and hip flexors, but also has activation of the knee flexors and ankle dorsiflexors. Transitioning the body weight from back onto the noodle to forward is mostly due to contraction of the trunk flexors and stabilizers. Extending the legs out behind the body is a contraction of the hip and knee extensors. It is important to maintain a strong contraction of the abdominals to avoid significant arching of the back.

The Bell with an Extension

Helps coordination, increases flexibility of back muscles and hips. Strengthens abdominal muscles and shoulders. Improves body alignment and posture. Stretches legs and lower back.

This exercise is the same as The Bell. The motion behind the torso is different.

This exercise begins with the legs and ankles held together in front of the torso. The knees are bent; the right foot is crossed over the left ankle to help keep the knees together.

The knees with the crossed over ankle are pulled forward to the water's surface.

Then the knees are pulled under the torso and the legs are stretched out.

The motion of forward with the knees followed by backward behind the torso is continued for 6 times.

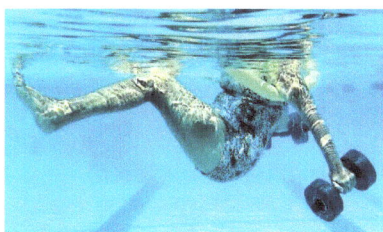

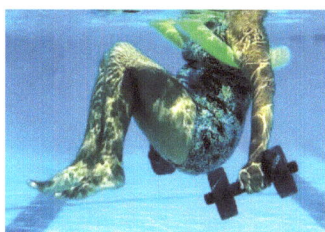

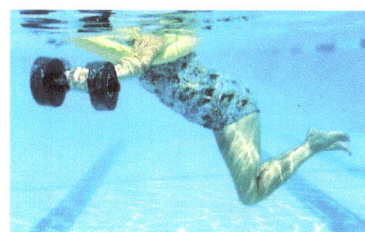

Continue the exercise by crossing the left foot over the right ankle and repeat the movement 6 more times.

To complete this exercise, stretch the legs out in front and bring feet to the surface of the pool.

ACTION: This exercise requires activation of the same muscles as previously described in "The Bell"; however, due to the crossing of the ankles, there is more demand on the hip adductors to bring one leg over the other as opposed to just bringing them together.

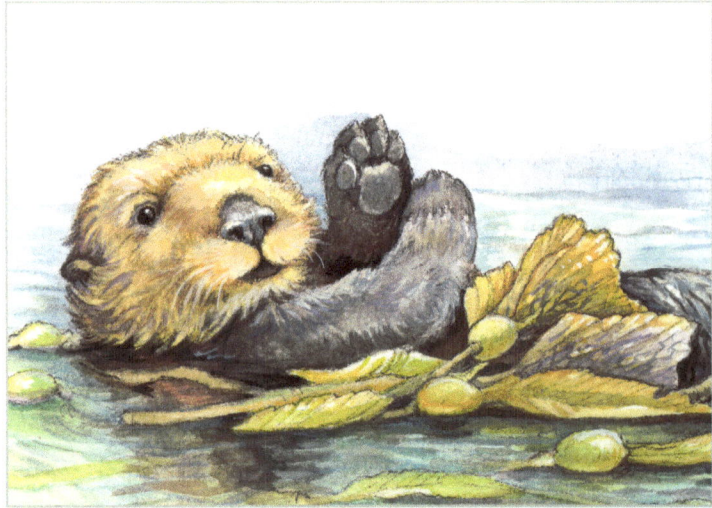

THURSDAY

"*I have severe arthritis, was very stiff, and was dealing with multiple joint pain issues. Water aerobics with Marti has been a godsend for my body. I could never do any of these exercises out of the water. I feel much better and stronger.*" – Joan B.

Thursday Pre-Exercise Muscle Information

NOTE: The wall exercises are NOT recommended for anyone who has had a back injury, back surgery, or troubles with the hips, including surgery.

Thursday's exercise routine involves shallow end, deep water, wall, and balance exercises.

After a warm-up session, the weights are placed along the pool edge, and replaced with a small diameter noodle for a few of the exercises. Then, the weights are again reused with the noodle for the duration of the session.

Stay in shallow water for several exercises and then move to the deep water to "hang out."

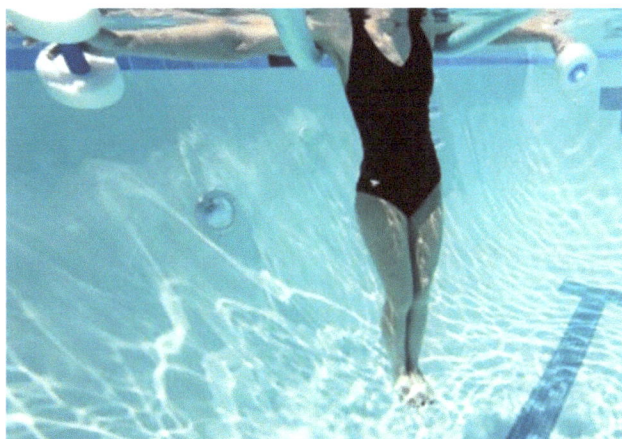

The body is supported by a noodle held under the shoulders/upper arms. The toes and feet are flexed or held naturally, below the torso. The arms remain on the "skinny" noodle or held out to the side with elbows bent. The body weight to hold the noodle in place behind the back comes mainly from the muscles in the lower back and from the lower arms. The position should be a relaxed one. In between each exercise in this section, the body "hangs out" for 30 to 60 seconds. The chin should be as parallel to the pool floor as possible to help stabilize the neck. This stabilizing movement is essential to the elevation of the arms.

Pedal or bicycle from the deep water to the edge of the pool for the wall exercises found in this section. The final exercises for Thursday's session are completed in the shallow end of the pool.

The "hanging out" position results in a stretching of the Latissimus Dorsi and Erector Spinae. At any time during any exercise the feet which the feet are firmly planted upon the pool floor, the following muscles are recruited: Gastrocnemius, Soleus, hamstrings, Iliopsoas, and the abdominals.

Ankle Pointy Toes

Helps alignment of the torso by strengthening the spinal muscles. Stretches the ankles and Achilles' tendon. Improves foot and leg strength.

Hang out with the noodle and weights in deep water. Hold knees and ankles together.

Point both toes down to the bottom of the pool; then, point both toes up. The pointing of down/up with the toes is one repetition and continues for 12 to 15 times.

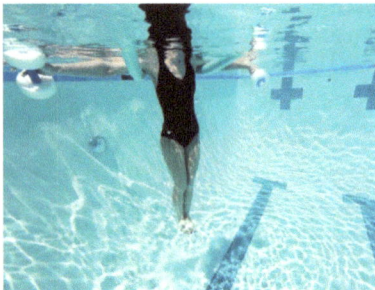

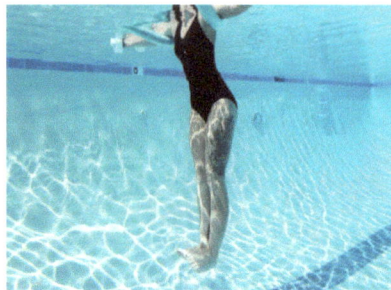

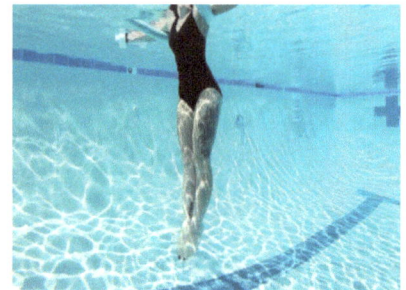

Then the person "hangs out" and rests until the next exercise.

ACTION: The "hanging out" position is mostly obtained by the buoyancy of the water on the noodle and weights holding the body up. There is a moderate isometric contraction of the shoulder adductors, but not as strongly as when the body is in the semi-reclined position. Holding the legs together requires constant contraction of the hip adductors. This exercise mainly targets alternating strengthening of the ankle dorsiflexors (bringing the toes up) and ankle plantar flexors (pointing the toes down).

Flat Feet to Alternating Sides

Helps with flexibility of the lower, internal back muscles. Stretches pelvic muscles and increases range of motion of the lower back, helping stability.

Remain in the "hanging out" position with the noodle at the deep end of the pool. Knees and ankles are held together. The feet are flat.

Very slowly, turn both flat feet to the right; then, very slowly turn them to the left.

Both flat feet are alternately turned right/left for a total of no more than 6 to 8 times (3 or 4 to the right; 3 or 4 to the left).

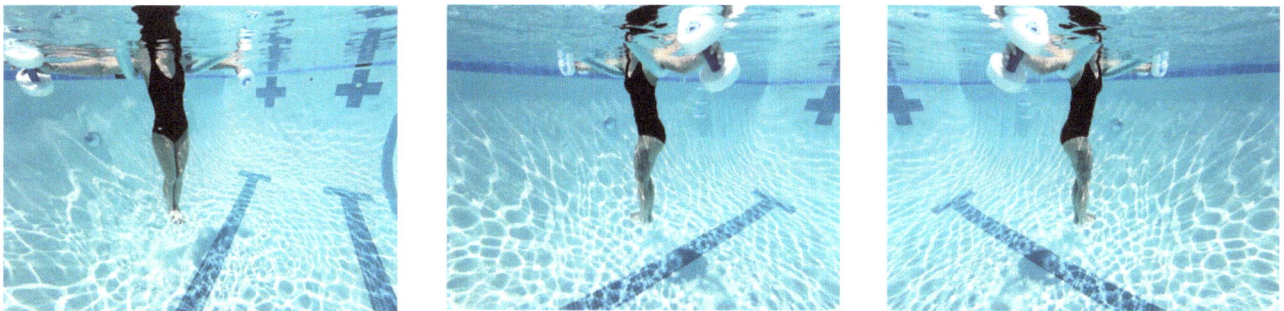

Hang out and rest until the next exercise.

ACTION: Keeping the body upright with legs together requires contraction of the trunk and pelvic stabilizers as well as the hip adductors. Keeping the feet flat is a constant contraction of the ankle dorsiflexors. Turning the feet to the right primarily involves activation of the right trunk rotators as the entire body is moved as a single unit, not just the feet turning. Because the body is moved as a unit together, there is added challenge on the scapular stabilizers to make sure the arms can maintain their position out to the side of the body and provide a stable base for the abdominal muscles and upper extremity muscles to anchor to.

Nordic Skier
(A Deep-Water Exercise)

Helps flexibility, coordination, range of motion, and body stability. Stretches pelvic area.

Remain in the "hanging out" position at the deep end of the pool. Hold knees and ankles together as if in a standing position. The soles of the feet are held flat.

The person moves the legs backward and forward, like a large scissor, keeping the feet flat. The scissor movement is repeated 20 to 25 times. One back and forth movement is counted as one repetition.

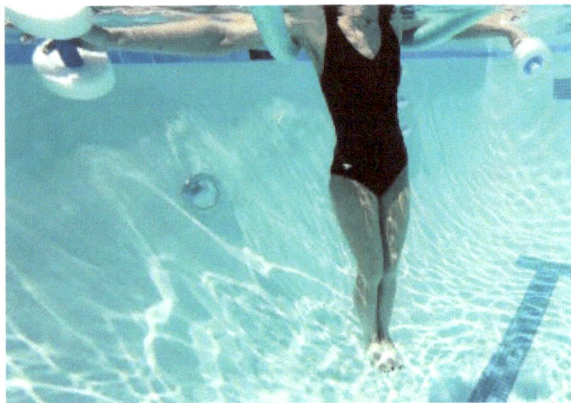

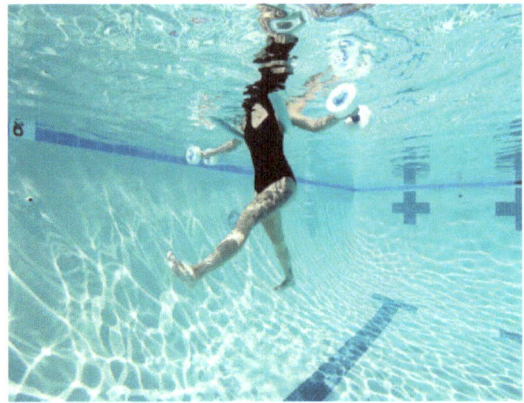

Then, the person "hangs out" and rests until the next exercise.

ACTION: As in the previous "hanging" exercises, the trunk and pelvic stabilizers must be active along with the hip adductors and ankle dorsiflexors to keep the legs together and feet flat, respectively. Moving one leg forward requires activation of the hip flexors, knee extensors and ankle dorsiflexors while moving the other leg requires activation of the hip extensors, knee extensors and ankle dorsiflexors. It is important to maintain pelvic and trunk stability throughout this exercise to avoid trunk rotation from side to side.

Ankle Circles

Helps coordination and strengthens small leg muscles. Improves body stability. Strengthens ankles and feet.

Hang out with the noodle and weights at the deep end of the pool. The legs are separated into the shape of a capital letter A and held shoulder distance apart. The ankles of both feet are circled inward 20 to 25 times. The circles should be kept small, about the size of the rim of a coffee cup.

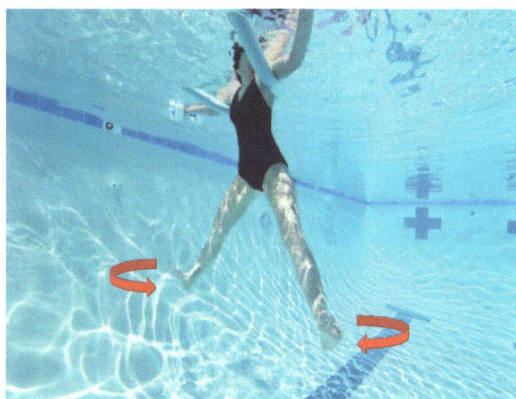

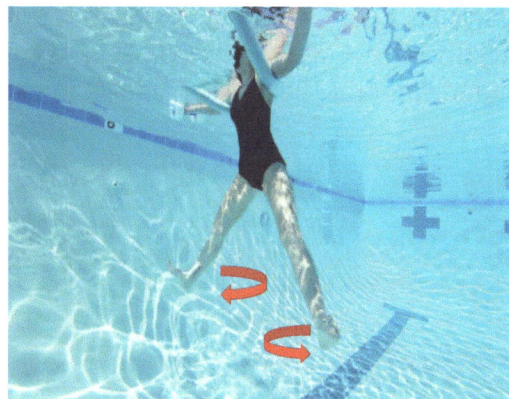

Next the ankles are circled outward 20 to 25 times. The circles should be kept small, about the size of the rim of a coffee cup.

ACTION: To obtain the starting position with the body "hanging" and legs making the "A" shape, the trunk and pelvic stabilizers must be active along with the hip abductors. The circular motion of the ankles is a sequential activation of the ankle dorsiflexors, ankle inverters, ankle plantar flexors and ankle evertors. Because the circular motion covers all movements of the ankles, this exercise is great for overall ankle stability.

Scissor Leg Stretch

NOTE: The exercise is repeated only three times.

Helps coordination, balance, pelvic stability. Stretches leg tendons and muscles, and Achilles tendons. Improves posture.

Hang out with the noodle in the deep water. Keep knees and ankles together.

The right leg with a flat foot is pulled/slides forward; the left leg with a flat foot is pulled/slides backward, making a big scissor with the legs. The feet are held flat. The toes on both legs are pulled upward and held for 30 seconds. Then, the legs are brought down to the "hanging out" position.

The left leg is pulled forward with a flat foot; the right leg with a flat foot is pulled/slides. Once again, make a big scissor with the legs, feet held flat. The toes on both legs are pulled upward and held for 30 seconds. The exercise is repeated right leg forward, flat feet and toes up; left leg forward, flat feet and toes up only three times.

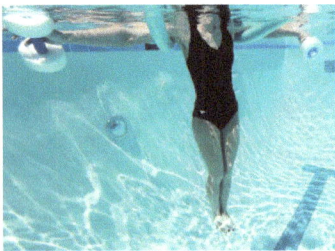

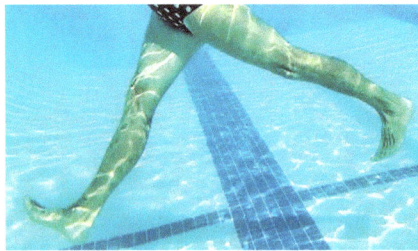

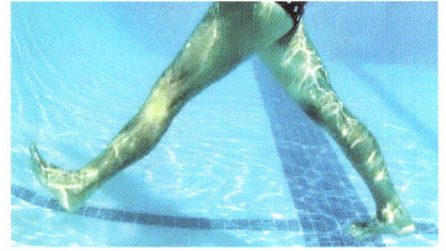

ACTION: Getting into the starting position for this exercise mostly utilizes the buoyancy of the water, noodle, and weights, but also requires engagement of the trunk and pelvic stabilizers and shoulder adductors throughout the exercise to maintain an upright trunk position. Pulling the left leg forward activates the hip flexors and knee extensors and pulling the toes upward engages the ankle dorsiflexors. Pushing the right leg back engages the hip and knee extensors while bringing the toes upwards engages the ankle dorsiflexors. This position primarily stretches the left hamstrings and calf muscles and the right hip flexors and calf muscles.

Slow Bicycle

Helps flexibility, range of motion of knees, ankles, and legs. Strengthens the pelvic area. Stretches lower back.

Hang out with their noodle in deep water. Keep knees and ankles together.

The right knee is pulled up to a 90-degree angle, the leg is stretched out, and the right leg is pulled back down to the starting position. The leg is pulled down forcefully by using the heel of the right foot.

The left knee is pulled up to a 90-degree angle, the leg is stretched out, and the left leg is pulled back down to the starting position. The leg is pulled forcefully by using the heel of the left foot.

This slow bicycle movement is alternated between right/left legs approximately 12 to 15 times.

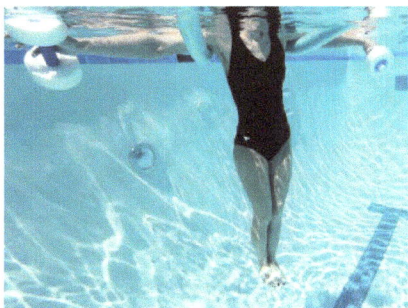

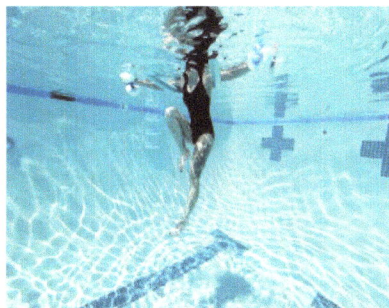

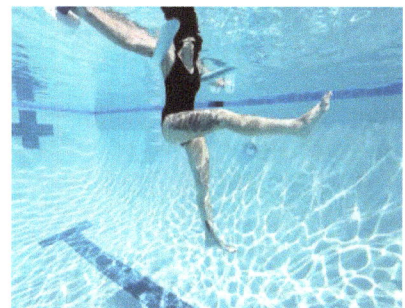

ACTION: Trunk and pelvic stabilizers and hip adductors are active to obtain the starting "hanging out" position with legs together. Lifting the knee to a 90-degree angle is primarily a contraction of the hip flexors and knee flexors. Stretching the leg out straight then utilizes the knee extensors, and pulling the leg forcefully back to the starting point with a straight leg requires mainly a contraction of the hip extensors. To keep the knee straight when pulling the leg back requires an isometric, stabilizing contraction of both the knee extensors and knee flexors to keep the knee from bending or hyperextending.

Knees to the Noodle

Helps knee, leg and hip flexibility. Strengthens and stretches lower body muscles. Enhances posture.

Hang out position at the deep end of the pool. Knees and ankles are held in the form of a capital letter A.

The person flexes both ankles and pulls both knees up to a 90-degree angle to touch the noodle, or as high as possible. The foot is held flat.

With feet held flat, push both legs simultaneously toward the bottom of the pool. Repeat this pull/push with knees, legs, and flat feet to the bottom of the pool 12 to 15 times.

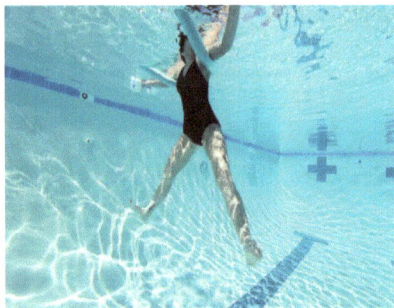

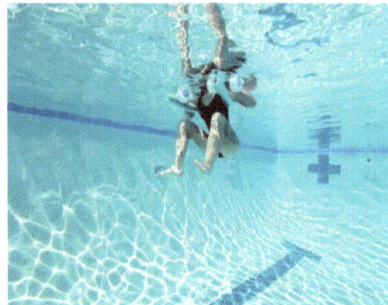

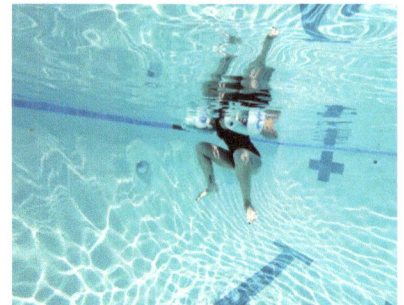

ACTION: To start in the "hanging out" position with legs in the shape of an "A," the trunk and pelvic stabilizers and hip abductors must be engaged. Pulling the toes up and "flexing" the ankles requires a contraction of the ankle dorsiflexors and pulling the knees up to the noodle uses the hip and trunk flexors with additional activation of the knee flexors. In this curled up position, the lower back should feel a nice stretch. When pushing the legs towards the bottom of the pool, a forceful contraction of the hip extensors and knee extensors is required. It is important to maintain a constant abdominal squeeze to avoid significant movement of the torso and isolate strengthening to the lower extremities and "core" musculature.

Butterfly Legs

Helps spinal alignment, increases flexibility. Stretches and strengthens pelvic muscles.

Holding knees and ankles together, assume "hanging out" position with the noodle at the deep end of the pool.

Both knees are pulled up simultaneously to a 90-degree angle. The back straightens so that the person feels as if they are sitting in a chair.

Then the knees are pulled out to the side like the wing of a butterfly. This butterfly movement of the legs is repeated 20 to 25 times.

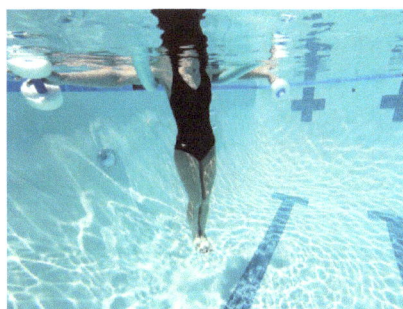

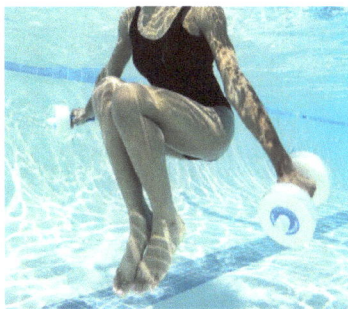

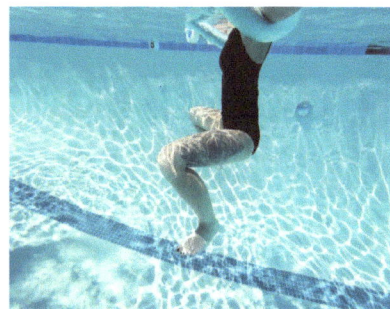

Then, the person "hangs out" and rests until the next exercise.

ACTION: The starting position requires contraction of the trunk and pelvic stabilizers, hip adductors and shoulder adductors. Pulling the thigh up to a 90-degree angle at the torso recruits the hip flexor and trunk flexor muscles, with the knees passively bending as the thigh raises. Straightening the back and maintaining appropriate posture requires stabilization of the core/abdominal muscles enabling the chest to remain upright. Pulling the knees out to the side engages the hip external rotators and keeping the knees bent will require engagement of the knee flexors. As the legs begin to move simultaneously, there is more demand put on the trunk and pelvic stabilizers to keep the torso still.

"Froggy" Pendulum
(A Three-Step Exercise)

Helps knee and hip flexibility, improves coordination and balance. Stretches and strengthens lower back and lateral (side) abdominals.

Bring the legs and feet to the water's surface from the "hanging out" position. Bring soles of both feet together causing the knees to turn outward.

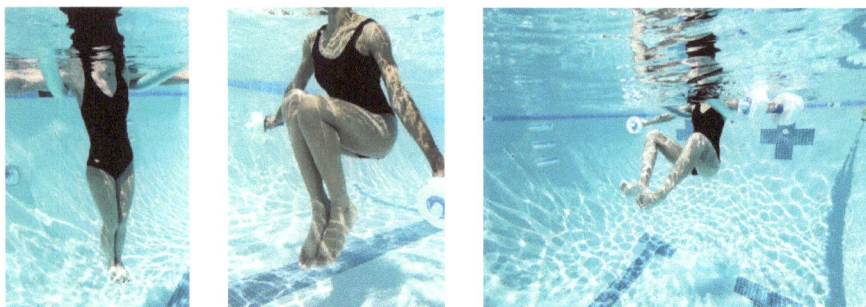

The soles of the feet are pulled into the torso and pushed back outward 12 to 15 times. Then the feet with soles together are pulled under the torso.

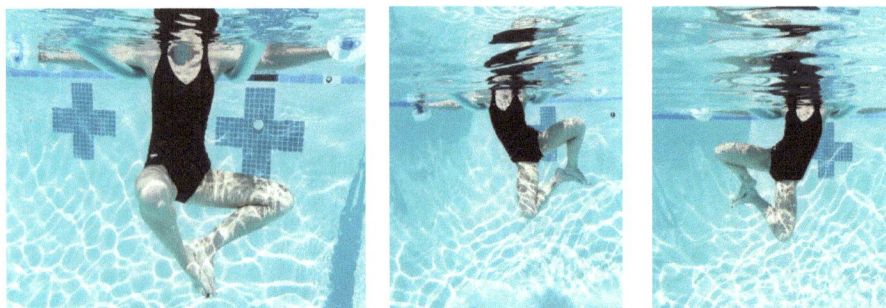

The knees are then pulled slightly inward keeping the soles of the feet together so that the lower back and pelvis area are not stressed. The feet with soles together are finally swung side to side, like a "froggy" pendulum. This "froggy" motion is repeated 12 to 15 times.

ACTION: Keeping the knees together in the starting position requires contraction of the hip adductors. The first step of this exercise is to bring the knees up to the chest from the "hanging out" position. This engages the hip and trunk flexors with passive bending of the knees. Bringing the soles of the feet together primarily targets the hip external rotators on both sides. The hip external rotators must remain active throughout the rest of the exercise to keep the knees apart. Pulling the feet in towards the torso engages the trunk flexors, hip flexors and knee flexors with constant contraction of the hip external rotators. Pushing the legs back out engages the trunk extensors, hip extensors, knee extensors, while keeping the hip external rotators engaged as well.

The third part of this exercise begins by bringing the legs back under the body into an upright position with the knees apart. This engages the trunk and pelvic stabilizers with additional activation of the hip external rotators. Swinging the legs from side to side engages the trunk side bending muscles. Bringing the right knee closer to the right shoulder is considered right trunk side bending and engages primarily the right internal and external obliques, and the quadratus lumborum muscles. Unlike the rotation motion at the torso, the internal and external obliques are activated on the same side with the side bend motion. The same action occurs on the left side. So while the right knee is brought towards the right shoulder, this is mainly strengthening the right side of the body.

Knees to the Wall with Noodle

NOTE: The wall exercises are NOT recommended for anyone who has had a back injury, back surgery, or troubles with the hips, including surgery.

NOTE: After this exercise and ALL remaining exercises for Thursday are to be done in the shallow end of the pool.

Helps to improve coordination, balance, posture and flexibility of lower body. Stretches the back.

NOTE: This is the beginning of a series of exercises, starting with showing the hand placement.

Pedal from deep water keeping the noodle still behind the shoulders to the wall. After grabbing the wall, pull the noodle with one arm and position it in front of the torso. The other arm holds onto the side of the pool.

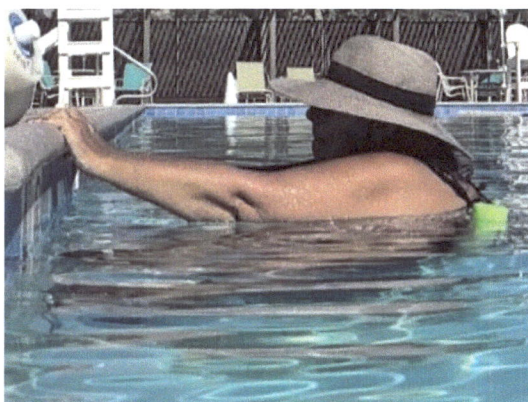

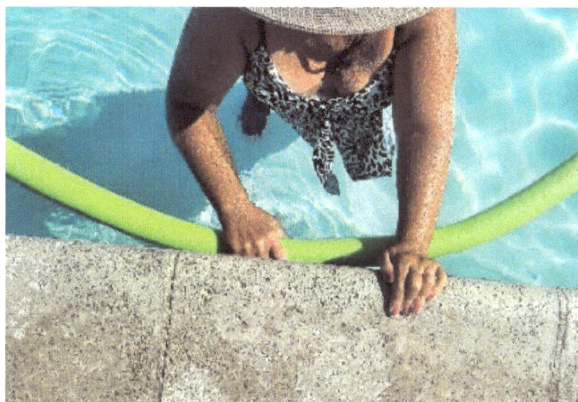

Place the noodle in front of the torso. Bring the knees to the side of the pool and push the noodle under one ankle at a time. Keep the ankles together. Then, place the knees on the pool wall, with the noodle remaining under the ankles. The arms are held straight. This position is maintained for 30 to 60 seconds.

ACTION: The main motion targeted in this transition is pushing the noodle down under the ankles. To push the noodle down against the buoyancy of the water engages the shoulder extensors, elbow extensors and wrist stabilizers. With the noodle under the ankles, the knees are being pushed into flexion and stretching the quadriceps. Pulling the knees to the wall engages the hip flexors and keeping the noodle under the ankles requires an isometric contraction of the ankle dorsiflexors.

Noodle at the Wall Knees Up

Helps to stretch and strengthen lower body, knees, feet, and legs. Improves spinal alignment.

Continue holding onto the wall and push the noodle downward using one hand at a time, one side at a time. First one heel and then the other heel is placed on the noodle.

The legs with heel placement form a capital letter A. Face the wall and keep back straight.

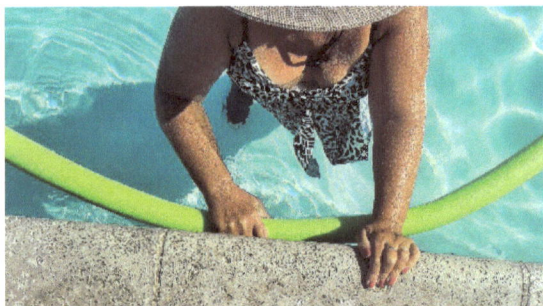

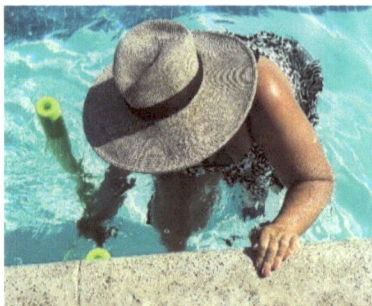

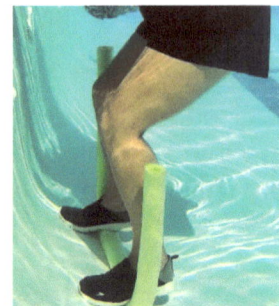

Push the noodle down with both heels to the starting position, legs straight and heels on the noodle. The buoyancy of the water will raise the noodle. (If the heels are not used and the feet are not flat, you will lose control of the noodle).

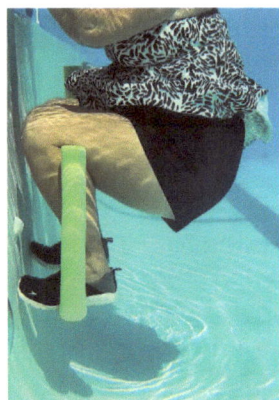

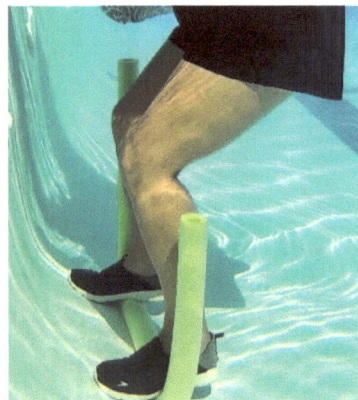

Repeat this downward/upward movement 12 to 15 times.

ACTION: In the starting position with legs straight and heels on the noodle, a constant stabilizing contraction of the trunk and pelvic stabilizers is necessary to avoid falling off the noodle. An eccentric contraction of the hip extensors, knee extensors and ankle plantar flexors is required to allow the noodle to rise in a controlled manner. Without the eccentric contraction of these muscles, the noodle would float to the surface of the water with no control and "pop" out of the water, throwing the body off balance. Slow, controlled movement is necessary when allowing the noodle to float up. Pushing the noodle back down involves activation of the hip and knee extensors to perform most of the motion. Both the ankle plantar flexors and dorsiflexors must be active to maintain balance on the noodle and keep the ankle steady.

Abdominal Work at the Wall

Helps lower body flexibility. Strengthens abdominals.

NOTE: <u>This is a very strenuous exercise</u>. It is NOT recommended for anyone with back problems, previous back surgery, or any medical problem. Don't forget to breathe!

Using the position from the previous exercise, the knees touch the wall. Push the legs out behind you so that the ankles rest on the noodle and the legs become straight on the noodle.

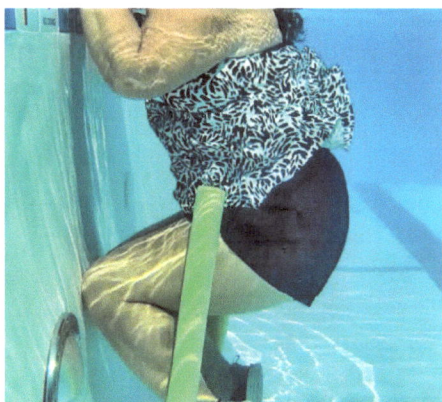

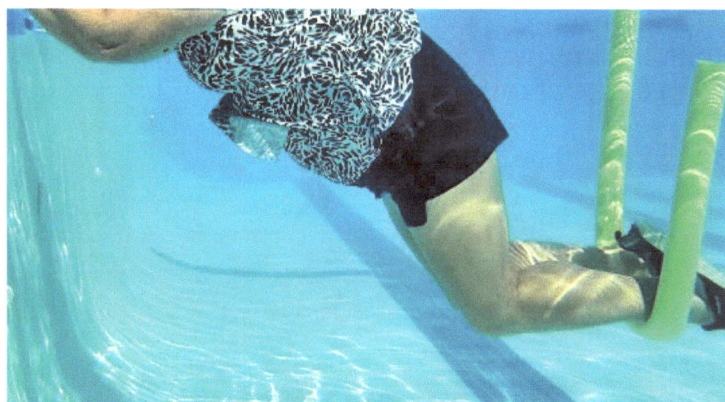

Curl the knees inward, and return the knees toward the wall, but without touching the wall. Arms bend slightly at the elbows. This pulling movement continues until you feels the noodle begin to slip. When the noodle begins to slip from the ankle, straighten the legs and push out again. Depending upon your strength, this push out and curl movement is repeated 15 to 20 times. The number of repetitions can be built up, starting slowly with 5 or 6 and moving up to a level you can easily achieve without overexerting yourself.

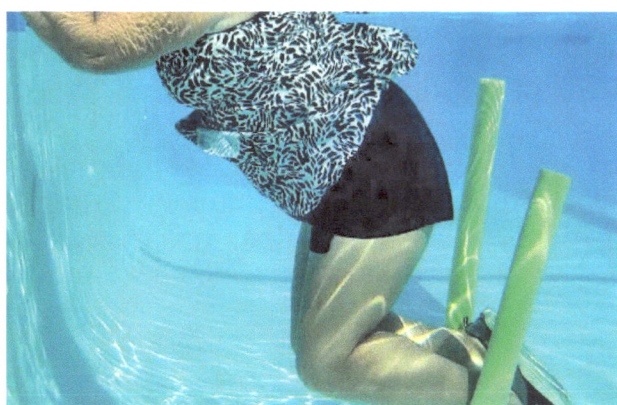

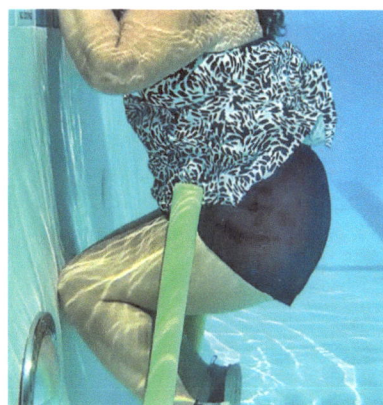

ACTION: This movement is accomplished by the water's buoyancy and the action of the Gluteus Maximus. The Quadriceps muscles push your leg straight behind the person. A contraction of the Latissimus Dorsi, Rectus Abdominus, transverse abdominus, and Multifidus muscles takes place with this movement. The Iliopsoas, Quadratus Lomborum and Anterior Tibialis muscles prevent the noodle from slipping out of position. The curling up motion is the action of the Iliopsoas and the Hamstring muscles.

Balancing on the Noodle at the Wall

Helps spinal alignment, posture, and flexibility. Strengthens hips, knees and lower back.

Hold onto the wall, and push the noodle downward using one hand at a time, one side at a time with one heel and then the other placing the heels on the noodle. First one heel and then the other placed on the noodle. The legs/heels make a capital letter A. Face the wall. Keep your back straight.

Let the buoyancy of the water raise the noodle; then push the noodle down with both heels to the starting position, legs straight and heels on the noodle. (If the heels are not used and the feet are flat, you will lose control of the noodle). This upward/downward movement is repeated for approximately 12 to 15 times.

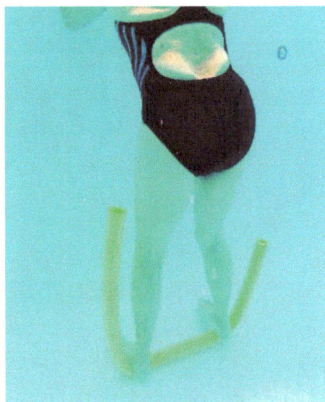

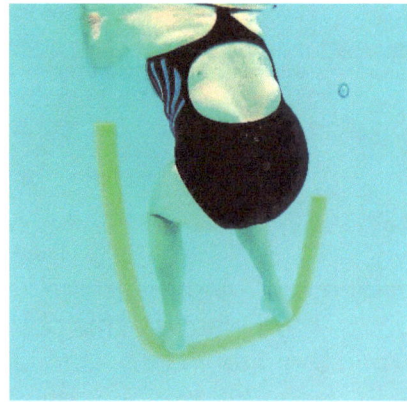

ACTION: In the starting position with legs straight and heels on the noodle, a constant stabilizing contraction of the trunk and pelvic stabilizers is necessary to avoid slipping off the noodle. An eccentric contraction of the hip extensors, knee extensors and ankle plantar flexors is required to allow the noodle to rise up in a controlled manner. Without the eccentric contraction of these muscles, the noodle would float to the surface of the water with no control and "pop" out of the water, throwing the body off balance. Slow, controlled movement is necessary when allowing the noodle to float up. Pushing the noodle back down involves activation of the hip and knee extensors to perform most of the motion. Both the ankle plantar flexors and dorsiflexors must be active to maintain balance on the noodle and keep the ankle steady.

Leg Stretch/Push Out from the Wall

Helps strengthen ankles, knees, and hips. Stretches lower body and legs.

NOTE: Avoid this exercise if you have had any type of hip replacement.

To begin this exercise, put both hands on the wall and place the noodle under your shoulders. Place toes of both feet on the wall between bent elbows.

The knees bend and curl upward toward the torso. The toes and hands remain on the wall. The knees are then straightened you push away from the wall with straight legs and straight arms. Hands hold the wall.

Hold "stretched out" leg position for <u>about 30 seconds</u>. Repeat only 3 times.

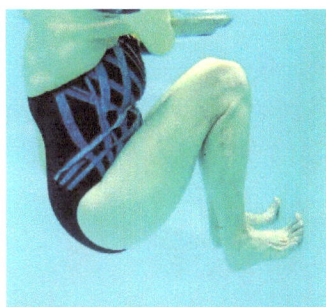

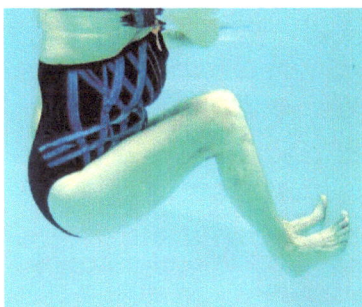

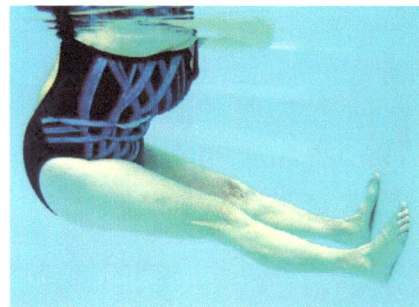

ACTION: To obtain the starting position, the trunk stabilizers and shoulder adductors must be active to keep the body afloat. The wrist stabilizers and finger flexors must also engage to hold onto the wall and support the body. Lifting the legs to the wall engages the hip flexors and ankle dorsiflexors. Straightening the legs out primarily engages the knee extensors. Holding this position provides a hamstring stretch that one should feel at the backs of their thighs.

Straight Leg, Flexing and Balancing

Helps flexibility, improves balance and spinal alignment. Strengthen legs and knees.

The right leg, held straight, is placed in the horseshoe-shaped noodle at the water's surface. The foot is held flat, toes pointing upward. The right toes are pointed and flexed 4 times.

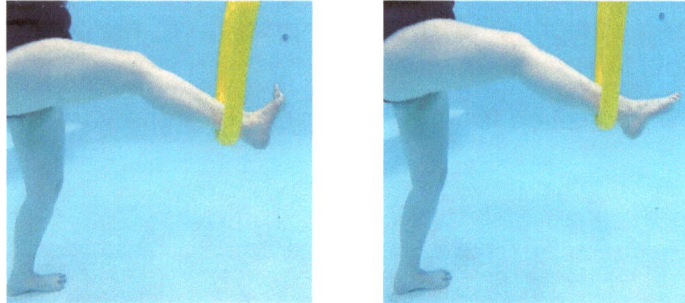

The straight right leg is then pulled downward and upward about 4 to 6 inches. Repeat this downward/upward movement 12 to 15 times.

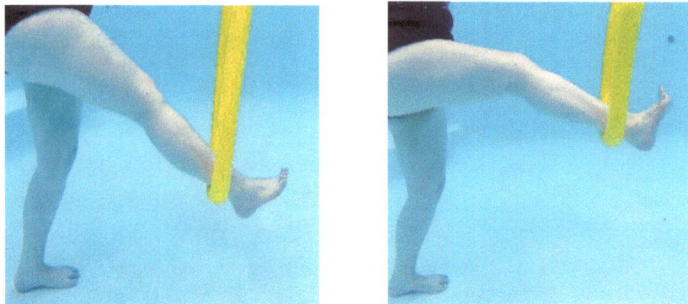

Repeat this exercise with the left leg.

ACTION: Turning the noodle upward into a horseshoe shape results in a contraction of the forearm pronators and the horizontal shoulder adductors. The stance stability is attained by a leg contraction of the hip adductors/abductors, and trunk and pelvic stabilizers. Lifting one leg into the horseshoe requires contraction of the hip flexors and knee extensors to straighten the leg. An isometric contraction of the knee flexors is necessary to keep the leg from floating to the surface. The pointing and flexing of the toe is an alternating contraction of the ankle dorsiflexors and ankle plantar flexors. Pulling the straight leg down and up after the four repetitions of the ankle pump is primarily an alternating pattern of concentric and eccentric contractions of the hip extensors. To pull the leg down is a concentric, or shortening, contraction of the hip extensors, and allowing the leg to float back up towards the surface in a controlled manner is an eccentric contraction of the same muscle group.

Balancing with Knee
(This is the second part of the series of exercises and is a continuation of the previous exercise)

Increases hip strength and flexibility. Strengthens lower abdominals, lower back and pelvic muscles.

The horseshoe-shaped noodle is pulled from a straight leg position, slips and is placed under the right-bent knee.

Push the right knee downward about 6 to 8 inches. The water's buoyancy allows the noodle to return to the water's surface. Repeat 12 to 15 times.

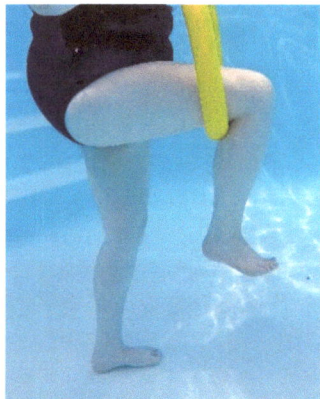

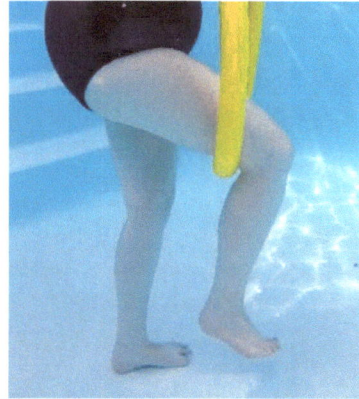

Repeat this exercise with the left knee.

ACTION: This exercise is primarily targeting the hip extensors. The hip extensors are located at the back of the hip and form the buttock muscles. When pushing the noodle down, the hip extensors are performing a concentric, shortening contraction and will feel like a tightening of the glutes. When allowing the noodle to slowly float back up, these same muscles are performing a lengthening, eccentric contraction. It doesn't feel the same as tightening up the muscle, but it is still being used to control the ascent of the noodle and avoid it "popping" back up to the surface.

Balancing Using Foot/Ankle

Helps balance and body stability as a straight spinal alignment is held. Strengthen knee and hip. Increases flexibility.

NOTE: Avoid this exercise if you've had any type of hip replacement. No greater than a 90 degree flexion at the affected hip.

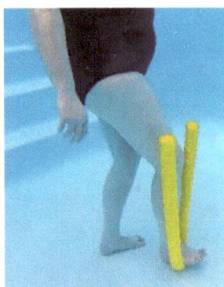

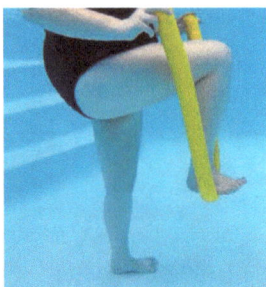

This is the last of the three exercises for balancing. Push the noodle downward so that the arch of the foot is centered on the middle of the noodle. Push the bent noodle to the bottom of the pool. Repeat 12 to 15 times.

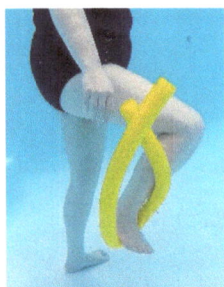

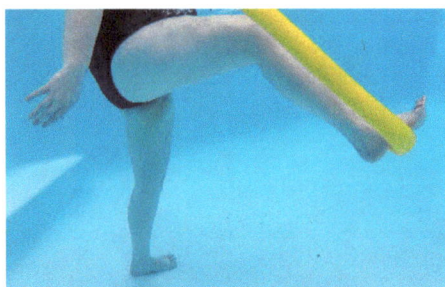

Then, the bent knee with the foot in the horseshoe-shaped noodle is turned to the right. Do not change the foot position on the noodle. The heel is pushed outward; the toe is pulled inward. Repeat 5 to 6 times.

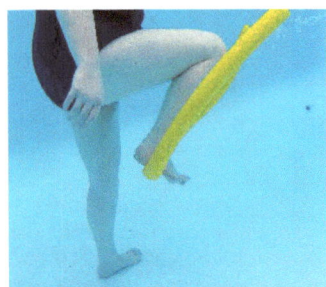

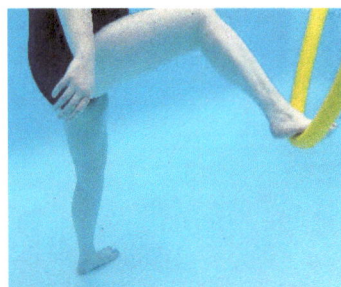

Then, place the right leg toward the front of the torso keeping the knee bent and the horseshoe-shaped noodle in the same position. Push heel outward and pull toe inward with the noodle is front of the torso. Repeat pushing/pulling movement 5 to 6 times.

Repeat this exercise with the left leg.

ACTION: This exercise is performed in a single leg stance position, which will challenge the pelvic stabilizers, the standing leg's hip extensors, knee extensors and ankle stabilizers. All of these muscle groups must be active to maintain a strong stance to give the moving leg a solid anchor from which to generate power. The first phase of this exercise involves lifting the knee up and down with the noodle under the arch of the foot. Lifting the knee slowly is an eccentric contraction of the hip extensors and an isometric contraction of the knee flexors. Pushing the knee back down is a concentric contraction of both the hip and knee extensors. The next movements involve knee flexion and extension with different angles of hip rotation to point the toes either towards the midline of the body, or out to the sides. When the toe is pointed in towards the midline of the body, the hip internal rotators are active. When the toe is pointed out to the side, the hip external rotators are active. Moving the foot out and back requires an eccentric and concentric contraction of the knee flexors.

Noodle Work for the Back

Strengthens arms, wrists, and hands. Stretches mid-torso abdominals and lower back.

This exercise requires a partner. One person holds their noodle stationary; the other person loops their noodle over their partner's noodle so that the noodle looks like a link of a chain.

Partners face each other. Keeping a firm grip on the noodle, each person lets their body fall backwards gently to their heels. Then return to the starting position. Repeat motion 25 times.

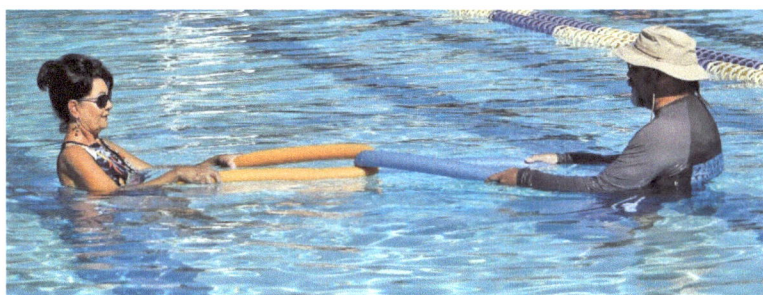

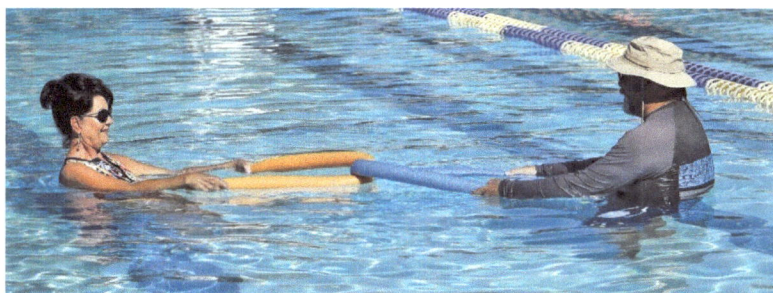

ACTION: "Falling backward" requires the muscles at the front of the ankle joint and arms to work against gravity, which is pushing the torso backwards into the water. These muscles must work to control the descent and avoid falling underwater. Recovering to the starting position is an effort of the arm, shoulder, and ankle muscles. The body begins its forward motion with activation of the scapular retractors. These muscles concurrently stabilize the scapula to allow the shoulder extensors and elbow flexors to generate force and bring the body back to the standing position. It is important to squeeze the abdominals throughout this exercise to keep the torso straight and stable.

Noodle Work for Shoulders and Arms

Helps coordination and shoulder flexibility. Stretches upper back and mid-torso muscles.

Working with a partner, pass one end of the noodle to your partner. Grab the end of your partner's noodle as your partner grabs the end of your noodle.

Each pushes and pulls the noodle back and forth. Repeat 25 times.

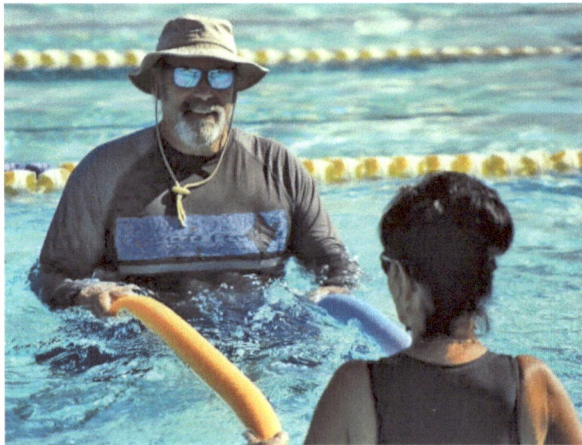

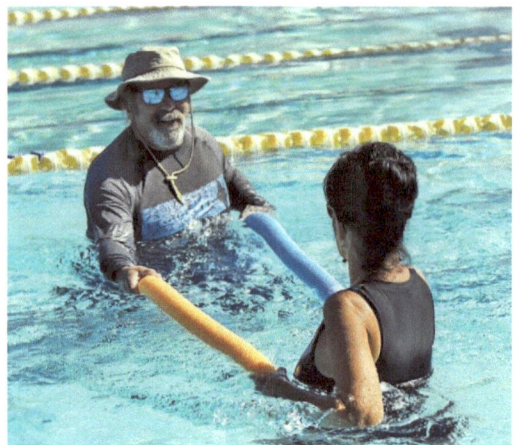

ACTION: Pushing the noodle forward engages the shoulder flexors and elbow extensors with coordination of the scapular stabilizers. There is an isometric contraction of the wrist and hand as the muscles maintain a firm grip on the noodle.

Pulling the arm /elbow behind the body engages the shoulder extensors and elbow flexors with contraction of the scapular stabilizers. There is a contraction of the wrist and hand muscles stabilizing the grip on the noodle.

Noodle Arm Exercises
(#1 and #2)

Helps increase shoulder and arm strength. Improves balance and posture and body alignment.

The noodle is held at each end. While jogging, bring the noodle ends together in front of the torso. Repeat the pulling in and pushing out 25 times.

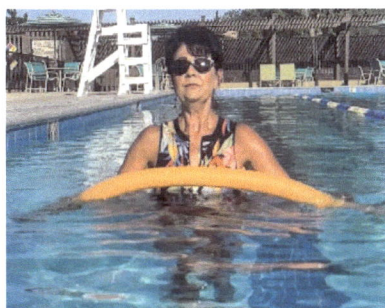

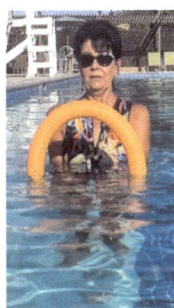

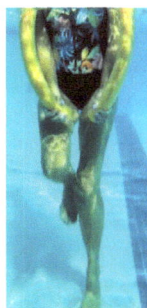

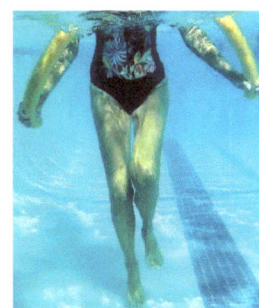

Then, place the noodle behind the torso. Continue jogging. Bring the ends of the noodle together behind the torso. Repeat 25 times.

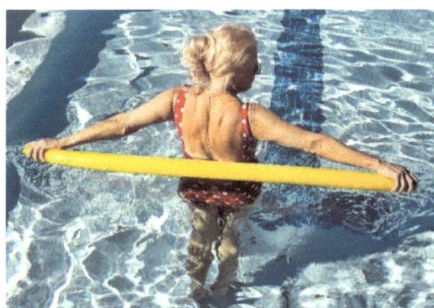

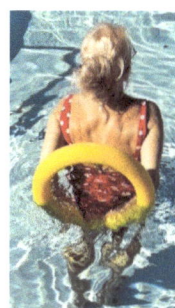

ACTION: Drawing the end of the noodle together in front of the torso engages the shoulder adductors and external rotators as well as the forearm supinators and elbow extensors. Keeping the scapular stabilizers engaged is important for the shoulder muscles to draw power from. Drawing the ends of the noodle together behind the torso is an action of the shoulder adductors and internal rotators as well as the forearm pronators. The controlled release of the noodle, in front and behind the torso, is an eccentric contraction of the muscles producing the action of the same muscles that draw the noodle ends together.

Pogo Stick with Variations

Helps balance, coordination, and agility. Increases knee and leg strength.

<u>Foot Placement</u>: Place the arch of the left foot on the noodle and push the noodle to the bottom of the pool. With an upward movement, the right arm pulls and slides the noodle upward. Using just the heel of the left foot on the noodle, place the toes of the left foot upon the pool floor. The heel of the right foot is then placed upon the noodle forming a capital letter A with the legs; the toes of the right foot are also placed upon the pool floor. Thus, both left and right heels are on the pushed down noodle; both sets of toes are on the pool floor.

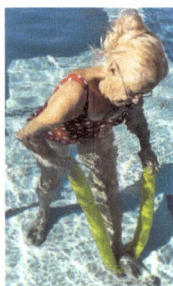

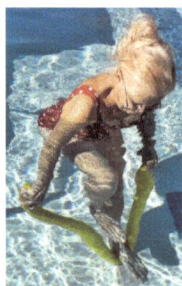

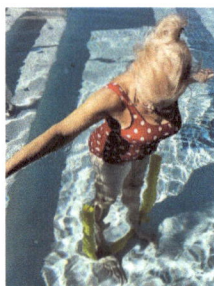

<u>Exercise</u>: Once you establish a firm, balanced position with both heels on the noodle and toes on the pool floor, the toes of both feet are lifted from the pool floor. Keep your balance and stand as straight as possible with both heels on the noodle. Then, jump up and down as far as possible while maintaining balance (as with a pogo stick).

<u>Extension of the exercise</u>: Jumping can be extended further by jumping in a circle to the left and to the right. You can also waddle forward and backward using the heels of the feet, slightly raising the knee, to establishing a balance position between the jumping and the waddling. It's fun!

ACTION: Obtaining and maintaining balance on the noodle requires coordination of the trunk and pelvic stabilizers as well as all the muscles of the legs and feet to keep the center of mass over a small target such as a noodle. Keeping the heels on the noodle and lifting the toes activates the ankle dorsiflexors, which will remain active isometrically throughout the exercise to keep the toes up. Jumping requires a quick, forceful contraction of the hip extensors and knee extensors.

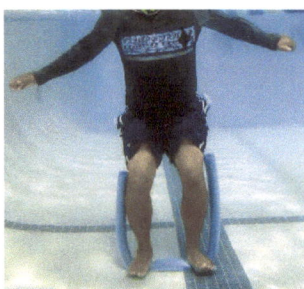

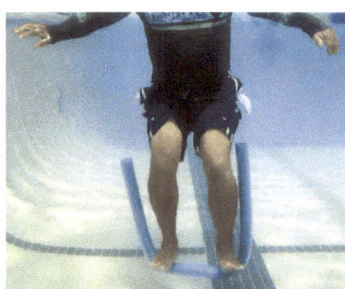

ACTION: Waddling on the noodle requires activation of the same stabilizing muscles to maintain balance on the noodle. Keeping the toes up position also requires an isometric contraction of the ankle dorsiflexors throughout. To step forward on the noodle, the hip flexors, knee extensors and ankle stabilizers must be active to lift and move the leg forward. This will further challenge your balance as you now have to maintain single leg stance position on a small noodle.

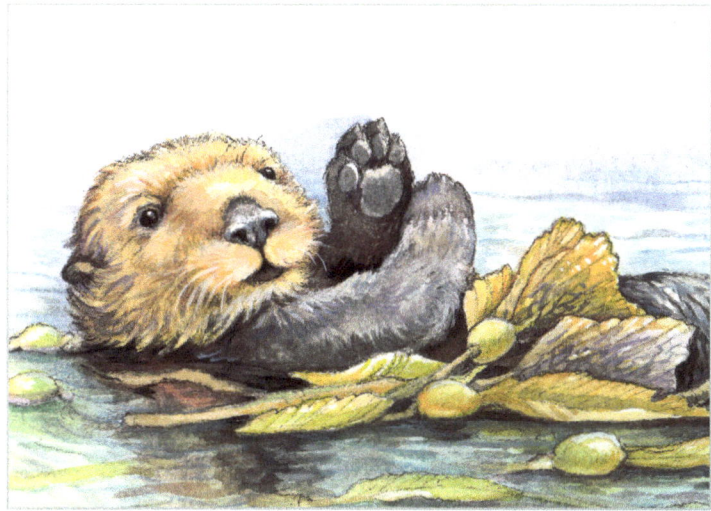

FRIDAY

"I am a ninety-three-year-old Christian woman. I don't get to escape to heaven until the Lord says "Come on Home!" Praise God for water aerobics. Marti, our instructor, loves aging people enough to coax us into strengthening our bodies. The water does its magic to soothe and heal. This gifted lady makes water exercise a time to build friendships as well as strengthen muscles." – Jo S.

Friday Pre-Exercise Muscle Information

The exercises for Friday are all therapeutic and slow moving exercises performed at the shallow end of the pool. They are designed to help with arthritis, pre- and post-surgeries, and other medical problems. The exercises are executed slowly and are designed to stretch the muscles, help the hip flexors, shoulder rotator cuffs, and inner body muscles.

Walking stretches the lower back, knee, ankles and pelvic muscles. Small motor muscles for posture and balance are all incorporated for a better total body movement.

Walking in water is ideal for arthritis. Walking backwards increases the circulation in the lower extremities. It is important to walk both forward and backward to change circulation and improve muscle movement.

In these exercises, stability is developed in the torso by having two feet placed firmly on the pool floor, which anchors the lower extremities (the legs) and gives support to the pelvis. When the pelvis is stable, the spinal and abdominal muscles, including the "core" muscles stabilize the torso. The torso being stable allows the scapula to transfer support to the upper extremities (the arms) by recruitment of the spinal scapular muscles and the scapular-arm muscles.

When squatting, the posterior pelvic tilt occurs because the digital attachment is anchored by the lower extremities (feet) placed on the floor of the pool, therefore moving the pelvis toward the legs. All muscles contract from both ends to the middle, attempting to bring the distal attachment, the end farthest from the center of the body, closer to the proximal attachment, the end closest to the center of the body. An example: In previous described exercises, the hamstrings were identified as knee bending muscles. In an exercise such as a squat, the hamstrings are pulling the proximal attachment at the pelvis. This motion of the pelvis is called posterior tilt. The determinant of stability is affected by either external or internal movement, proximal or distal.

Shoulder Rolls

Helps rotator cuffs in shoulder area. Relaxes upper back and neck.

Stand comfortably with feet placed firmly on the pool floor with arms at rest at the side of the body throughout the exercise. Both shoulders are pulled upward, toward the chin and jawline.

The shoulders are then "circled" pulling them forward slowly and around. Repeat this circular motion 12 to 15 times.

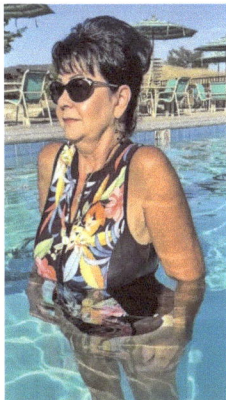

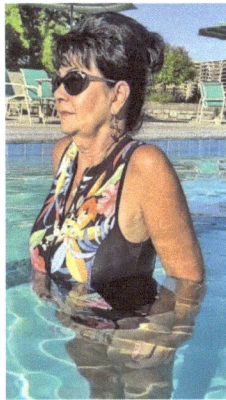

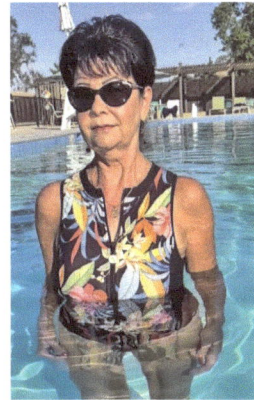

ACTION: Scapular elevation occurs when the shoulders are pulled upwards towards the ears and this engages the levator scapulae and upper trapezius muscles. Scapular protraction occurs when the shoulders are pulled forward and this is primarily performed by the pectoral muscles. The downward motion of the shoulders is scapular depression, which primarily engages the latissimus dorsi muscle. Moving the shoulders backwards is scapular retraction, which is mainly performed by the rhomboids and the middle trapezius. All of these muscles are engaged in sequence as the shoulders move in all directions to form a circle.

This motion is unique because the shoulder joint is not moving, but the scapula is moving on the posterior chest wall. Looking at the photo, #2 photo shows the elevation of the shoulder joint performed by scapular elevation.

Palms Together

Helps stretch shoulders and upper torso. Strengthens arms. Increases upper body flexibility.

Pull both arms up, puts both palms together and places them center front of the torso at the water's surface.

Both palms are pulled to the left and then to the right. Repeat this alternating movement 20 to 25 times.

NOTE: For this exercise, the shoulders should be below the water. The model was asked to show arms and hands placement above the water for a better understanding of the execution of the exercise.

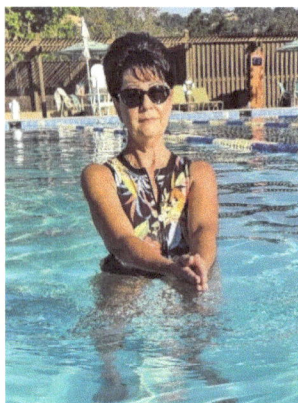

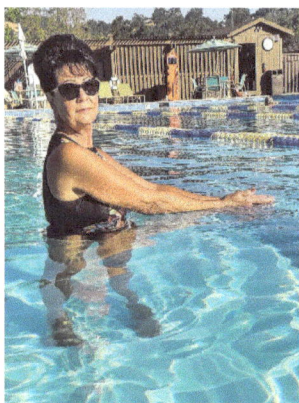

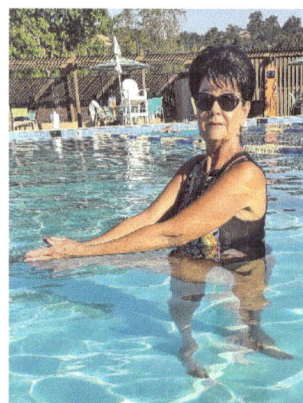

ACTION: Water buoyancy is the main force keeping the arms at the surface of the water, but the shoulder horizontal adductors must be constantly active to keep the palms together. Because the palms are held together, they act like a paddle in the water and increase the resistance and muscle challenge when performing the trunk twist. To twist from side to side, the trunk rotators must be engaged. Because of how the lateral trunk muscles are oriented, both sides of the body will be strengthened and stretched throughout the entire exercise.

Alternating Arm Pulls
(Photos show a seated position for more accurate arm movement)

Helps to strengthen arm control and shoulders. Stretches upper body muscles.

The palms from the previous exercise move to face downward toward the pool floor. Arms are shoulder distance apart.

The right flat palm is pulled down to tap the left thigh, then returned to the starting position.

The left flat palm is pulled down to tap the right thigh, then returned to the starting position.

Repeat this alternating movement 20 to 25 times. Each right/left movement counts as one repetition.

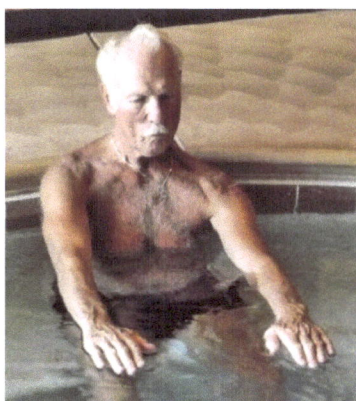

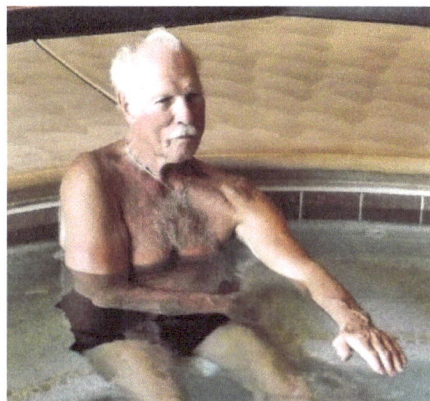

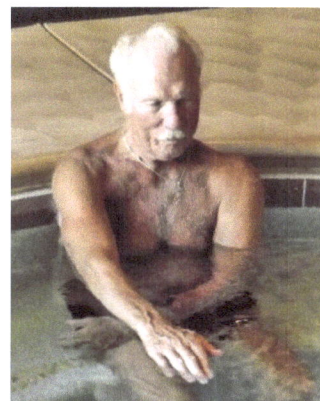

ACTION: Turning the palms downward engages the forearm pronators throughout the entire exercise. Keeping the palm face down and moving it downwards in the water increases the water resistance and muscle challenge. Bringing the arm down across the body to the opposite hip challenges the shoulder horizontal adductors, shoulder extensors and shoulder internal rotators. The scapular stabilizers must remain active throughout this exercise to provide a stable base for the shoulder muscles from which to generate force. When the hand is all the way down next to the hip, a stretching sensation can be felt along the top of the shoulder and in the mid back. The muscle groups in these areas include the shoulder abductors and scapular retractors.

Palms Down with a Push/Pull

Helps spinal stability. Stretches lateral (side) abdominal muscles. Strengthens arms, wrist, and hands.

The arms with flat palms are on the water's surface. Bend the elbows to align them with the shoulders. Push both flat palms downward (palms down) to your hips.

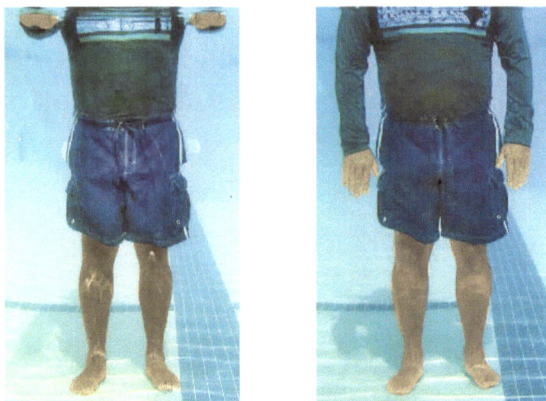

Flip your palms over (palms up) and pull them back up to the water's surface. Repeat this downward/upward movement 12 to 15 times. (The exercise motions are exaggerated for clarity.)

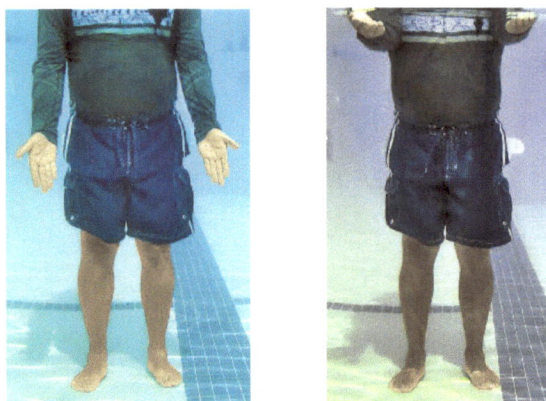

ACTION: Keeping the arms flat on the surface of the water engages the forearm pronators and shoulder internal rotators and pushing the arms down to the hips activates the shoulder extensors and elbow extensors. Flipping the palms up engages the forearm supinators and shoulder external rotators and lifting them back to the water's surface activates the shoulder flexors and elbow extensors. While pushing down, maintaining a steady trunk position requires a strong isometric contraction of the trunk and pelvic stabilizers.

Hands Up

Helps to strengthen and stretch upper back. Increases shoulder and spinal stability. Increases rotator cuff mobility.

Place the arms on the surface of the water; bend the elbows, lining them up with the shoulder, palms flat at the surface.

Raise the hands and hold for two seconds then push the hands back to the water surface.

Repeat this movement 12 to 15 times.

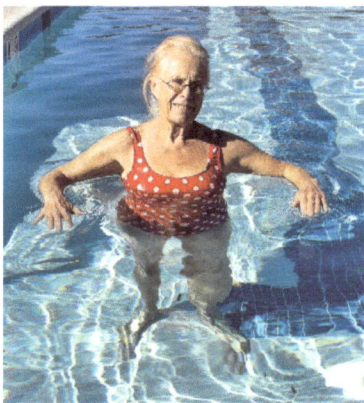

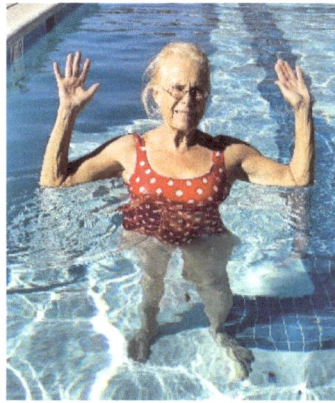

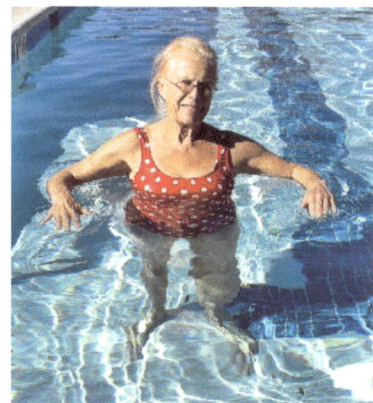

ACTION: To obtain the starting position, the shoulders must be abducted to 90 degrees, the elbows are flexed, and the shoulder internal rotators bring the forearms down to the surface of the water. The forearm pronators and wrist stabilizers are active to keep the wrists and forearms strong. Raising the hands up is primarily an action of the shoulder external rotators but the elbow flexors, forearm pronators and wrist stabilizers must be active isometrically to hold the bent elbow and neutral wrist position. Pushing the hands back down to the surface is an action of the shoulder internal rotators.

Elbow Pulls

Helps to strengthen shoulders and upper back and neck. Stretches upper back.

Elbows are bent and aligned with the shoulders. The hands are held upward.

The bent elbows are then pulled inward are far as possible and brought back to the starting point. Each inward/outward movement is counted as one repetition.

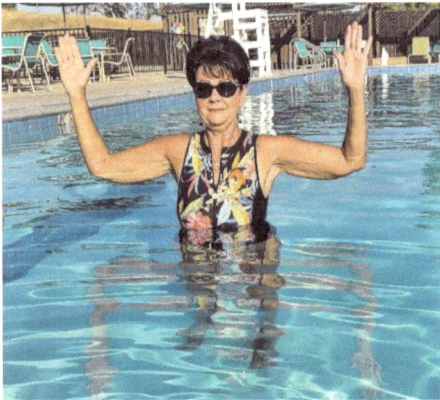

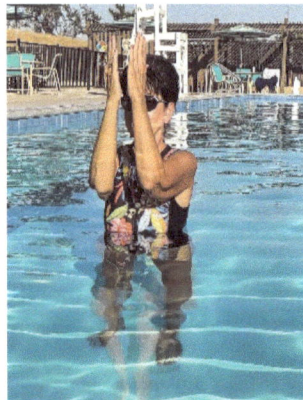

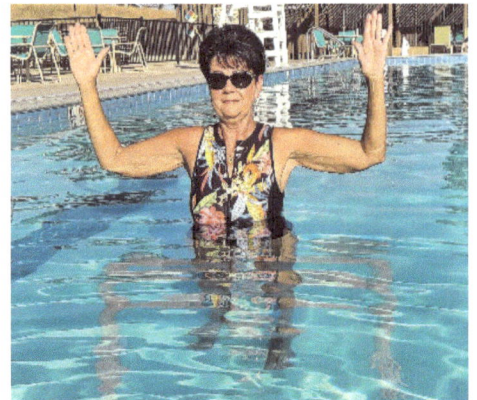

Repeat the inward/outward movement 12 to 15 times.

ACTION: Obtaining the starting position requires abduction of the shoulders to 90 degrees, external rotation of the shoulders to bring the hands up, elbow flexion to 90 degrees and pronation of the forearms. The action of bringing the elbows together in front of the body is called horizontal adduction of the shoulder. This movement is accomplished by the concentric contraction of the Pectoralis Major and minor muscles. The rotator cuff muscles remain isometrically active to keep the shoulder stable as it moves. An isometric contraction is performed when a muscle does not shorten or lengthen, but uses its strength to hold the same position to avoid being stretched. The scapula becomes protracted and pulled around the rib cage with a concentric contraction of the middle and lower Trapezius, and the Rhomboid muscles.

The return to the start position is an action called horizontal abduction. This movement is accomplished by a concentric contraction of the posterior Deltoid muscle, pulling on the scapula as it returns to its starting position. This movement is a concentric contraction of the rotator cuff muscles and scapulothoracic muscles.

The Archer
(Photos show a seated position for more accurate arm movement)

Helps to stretch shoulders and upper torso. Strengthens neck and arms. Aids spinal alignment and flexibility when standing.

Pull the palms together facing toward the left. Keep the palms flat with thumbs up.

Pull or draw the right palm, keeping the thumb upward, across the chest. Straighten the arm as it comes across the chest to fully extend it. Then pull the arm forcefully back toward the left palm. Repeat this motion 12 to 15 times. Switch sides and repeat this motion 12 to 15 times.

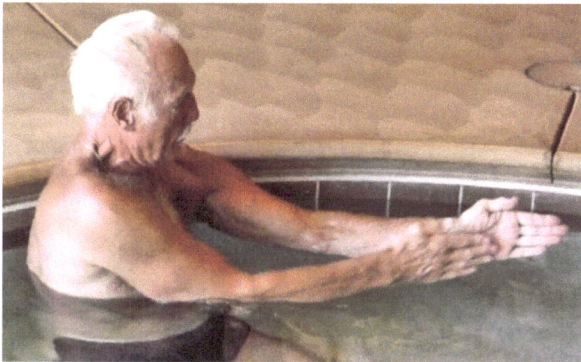

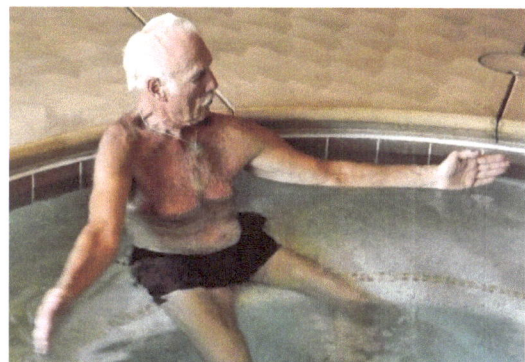

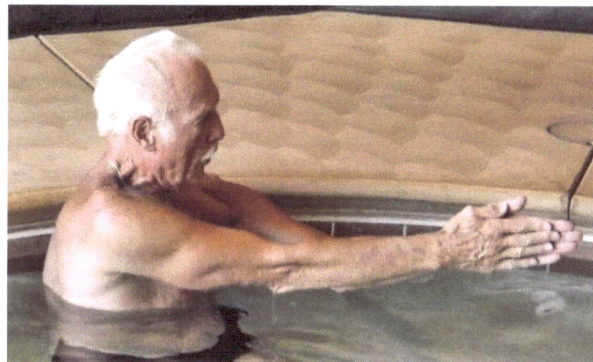

ACTION: This exercise starts with trunk rotation; arms held together and out in front of the body. This position activates the trunk rotators, elbow extensors and shoulder horizontal adductors. Drawing the arm across the chest engages the moving arm's elbow flexors, shoulder extensors, and scapular retractors while engaging the wrist and forearm stabilizers. Straightening the arm as it goes across the chest engages the elbow extensors and requires constant wrist stabilization to avoid having the hand flap in the water. To return to the starting point, the straight arm is drawn back to the midline of the body to meet with the other hand. Forcefully bringing the arm back requires a strong contraction of the shoulder horizontal adductors and elbow and wrist stabilizers.

The torso should remain facing the same direction throughout this exercise, which requires contraction of the torso and pelvic stabilizers. Without activation of these muscles, the trunk would rotate back and forth with the arm instead of maintaining a constant position.

Thigh Slides
(An Alternating Movement)

Helps to stretch upper torso. Increases flexibility of upper torso and lower back.

Stand comfortably in the water with feet firmly on the pool floor. Place palms beside the thighs.

Slide the right palm down the right thigh. Pull the right palm back and slide the left palm down the left thigh.

Repeat this sliding motion from right to left 12-16 times.

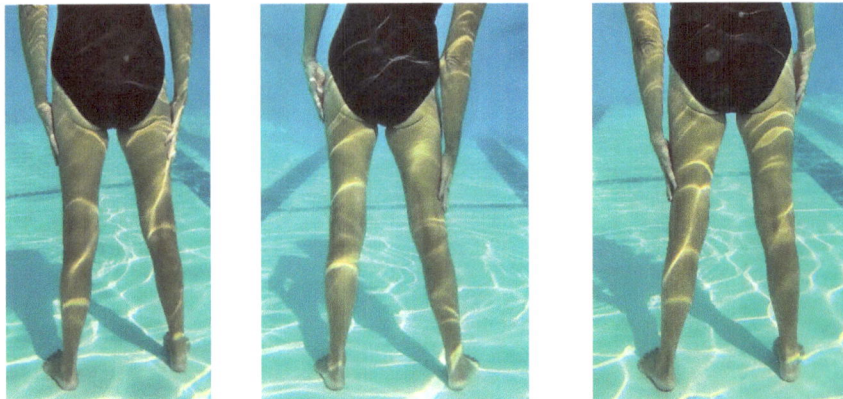

Then, the palms are <u>placed behind the thighs</u>. Slide the right palm down the back of the right thigh. Pull the right palm up and slide the left palm down the back of the left thigh.

Repeat the sliding motion down the back of each thigh 12 to 16 times.

ACTION: This movement is an action of the torso. As the palm reaches for the side of the knee, the lateral abdominal muscles act to laterally flex the torso and bring the arm down the side of the leg. If the right arm reaches down the right leg, the right-side abdominals are active and the left side is stretching. To stand back up straight, the left side abdominals must activate to pull the torso back to midline.

As the palms slide down the back of the thigh, the erector spinae muscles are drawing the torso backward and down in addition to the lateral abdominals that laterally flex the torso.

Arm Pull In/Push Out with a Squat

Helps coordination and balance. Strengthens knees and back.

Stand with feet flat on the pool floor. Legs are shoulder distance apart. The noodle, with arms/hands shoulder distance apart, is placed out and in front of the torso. Palms are facing downward on the noodle and the thumb and fingers grasp the noodle.

Draw the noodle inward and squat as the noodle comes inward to your chest; then, push the noodle back out and resume standing. Repeat 20 to 25 times.

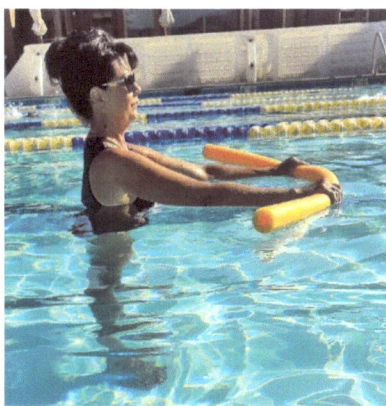

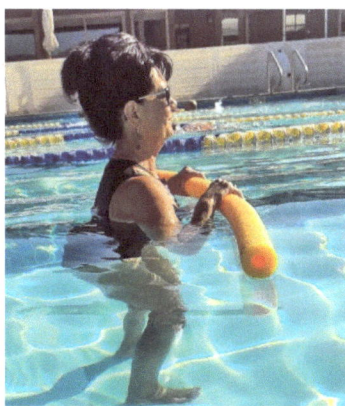

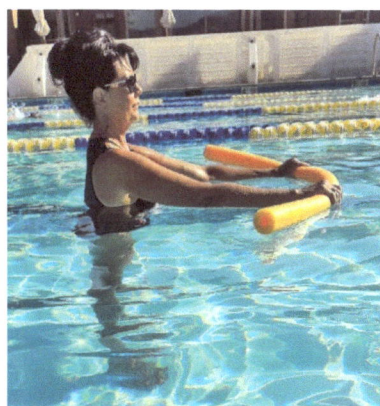

ACTION: Grasping the noodle with the palms downward and pulling toward the torso recruits the finger flexors, forearm pronators and elbow flexors. At the wrist, the muscles on top and bottom of the forearm are challenged to maintain stability. Pushing the noodle back in front of the body primarily engages the elbow extensors. The opponens pollicis is recruited using the thumbs to grasp the noodle.

To perform the squat, the torso and pelvic stabilizers must be active to keep the back straight throughout the exercise. Sitting back and down into the squat engages the hip extensors, knee extensors and ankle plantar flexors eccentrically to lower the body slowly into the water. To stand back up, these same muscles are activated concentrically to push the body back up against gravity, assisted by the buoyancy of the water.

99

Do Your Laundry

Helps strengthen arms, elbows, and shoulders.

The noodle is turned into the shape of a horseshoe. Then, the hands slide on the noodle to turn thumbs inward. Palms are rotated to face down toward the pool floor as the noodle is pulled close and next to the torso. The noodle is pushed up and down with palms down 20 to 25 times. The arms become straight each time the noodle is pushed down toward the hips, remaining close to the torso. The hands remain shoulder distance apart as you do your "laundry."

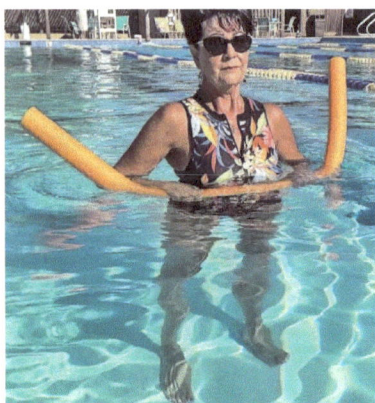

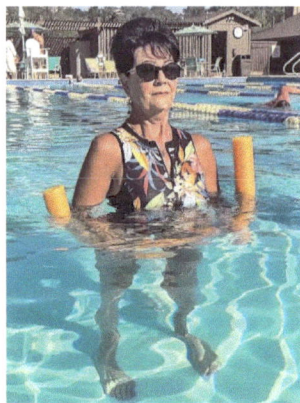

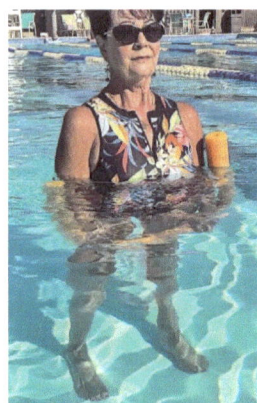

ACTION: Turning the noodle into a horseshoe shape and pushing the thumbs down towards the pool floor recruits the forearm pronators and shoulder internal rotators. Pushing the noodle down and maintaining this forearm position requires a concentric contraction of the elbow extensors and shoulder flexors with a maintained isometric contraction of the forearm pronators and shoulder internal rotators.

Bringing the noodle back to the top of the water requires an eccentric contraction of the elbow extensors and shoulder flexors to keep the noodle from popping back up to the surface, uncontrolled.

Scratch Your Back

Helps strengthen arms, elbows, and shoulders. Increases and creates a more upright posture.

The easiest way to get a good position is to briefly sit on the noodle before placing it behind the back. The noodle with palms and thumbs held downward to the horseshoe shape is close to the back. Arms and hands are next to the torso.

Resuming a standing position, a push/pull is the performed up and down the back. Keep the noodle as close to the back as possible.

Repeat this "scratch the back" 20 to 25 times before returning the noodle to the front of the torso.

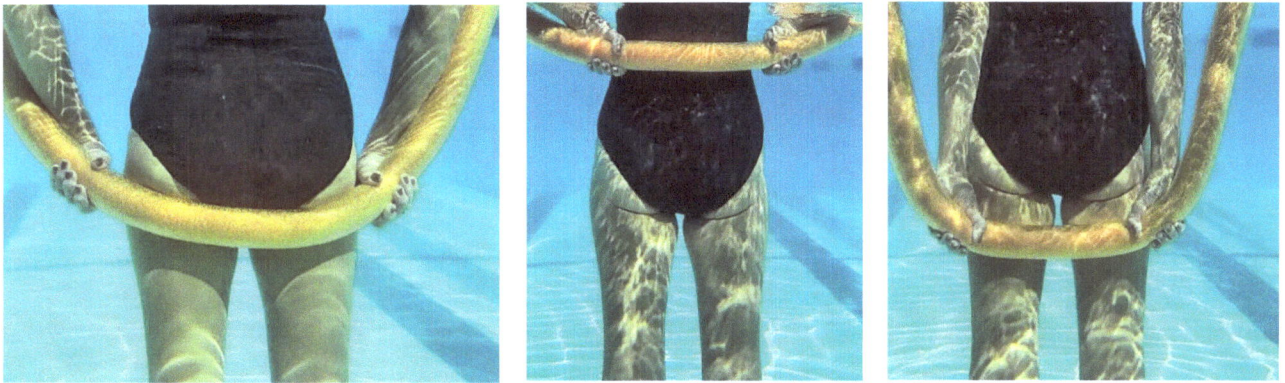

ACTION: To obtain the starting position with palms and thumbs held downward on the noodle with arms behind the back requires contraction of the forearm pronators, shoulder internal rotators, shoulder abductors, and wrist stabilizers. Pushing the noodle down involves contraction of the elbow extensors, shoulder adductors and the shoulder internal rotators. To keep the torso upright, it is important to squeeze the abdominals throughout the entire exercise. Bringing the noodle back up to the starting point involves an eccentric contraction of the same muscles used to push it down. They are performing a lengthening contraction to keep the noodle from popping up uncontrolled.

Side-to-Side

Helps strengthen spinal alignment. Stretches upper torso and neck.

Place noodle in front of the torso. Maintain the capital letter A stance with feet on the pool floor. Hands are moved as close to the end of the noodle as possible. Keep head straight ahead. Focus on an object across the pool from where you are standing.

The noodle is moved and turned from side to side/right to left from the torso without turning the head. Repeat 12 to 16 times.

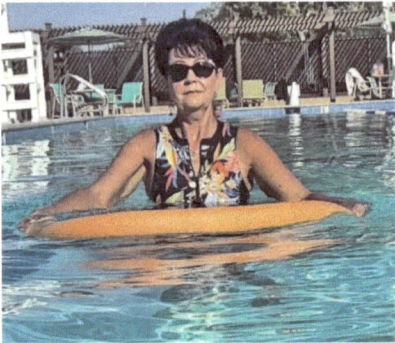

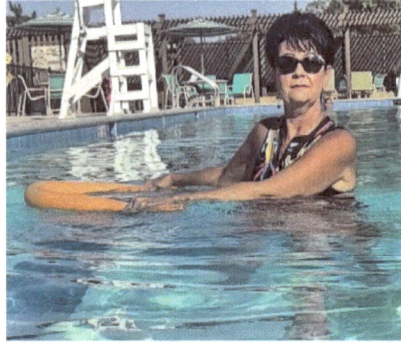

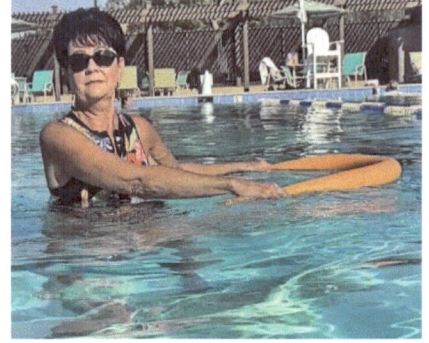

ACTION: To obtain the starting position with palms and thumbs held downward on the noodle with arms behind the back requires contraction of the forearm pronators, shoulder internal rotators, shoulder abductors, and wrist stabilizers. Pushing the noodle down involves contraction of the elbow extensors, shoulder adductors and the shoulder internal rotators. To keep the torso upright, it is important to squeeze the abdominals throughout the entire exercise. Bringing the noodle back up to the starting point involves an eccentric contraction of the same muscles used to push it down. They are performing a lengthening contraction to keep the noodle from popping up uncontrolled.

Pretzel with Straight Arms
(For a "skinny" noodle)

Helps strengthen lower torso, arms, and shoulders. Increases spinal stability.

The ends of the noodle are turned and tied into a pretzel shape. The "pretzel" is held downward. The hands grasp the ends of the noodle below the knotted part of the pretzel.

Keep feet and heels firmly planted on the pool floor.

The "pretzel" is first pulled down to the thighs and then back to the water's surface.

Pull up your toes if the heels seem to want to move upward.

The "pretzel" is pulled down and up in front of the torso 20 to 25 times. Then the pretzel comes to rest in front of you on the water's surface.

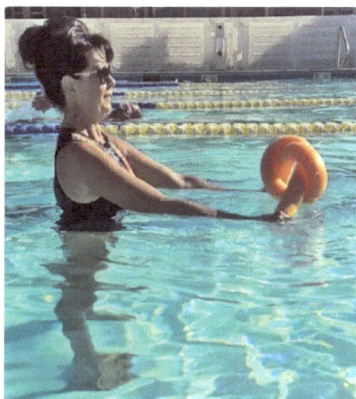

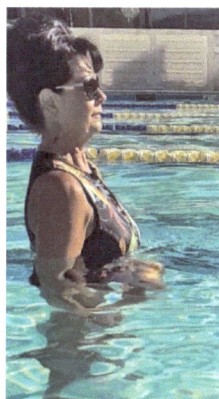

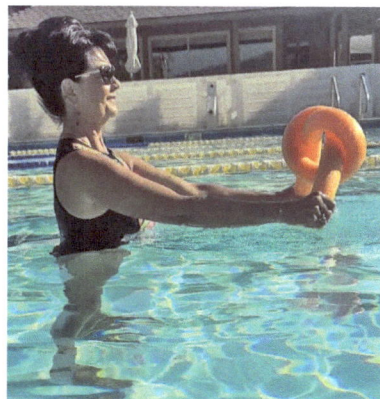

ACTION: Tying the noodle into a knot centralizes the mass of the noodle and increases the amount of water buoyancy experienced during the pushdown. Starting with the arms out straight engages the elbow extensors and shoulder flexors. Pulling the noodle down strengthens the shoulder extensors, elbow extensors and trunk stabilizers. Allowing the noodle to rise back to the surface results in an eccentric contraction of the previously mentioned muscles.

Side-to-Side Pretzel

Helps posture, balance, and spinal alignment. Strengthens elbows, arms, and upper torso muscles.

The noodle remains in a pretzel shape. Legs remain in a capital letter A. Feet are firmly planted on the pool floor.

The "pretzel" is held out in front of your torso at arm's length. The "pretzel" is pulled into the chest.

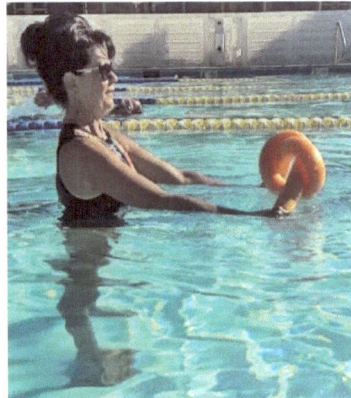

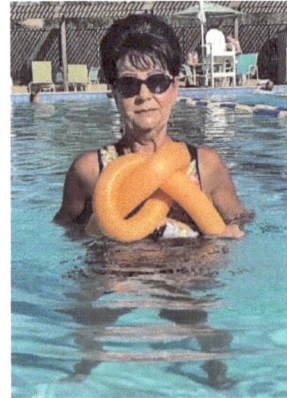

Then the "pretzel" is pushed to the left, pulled back to the chest, and pushed to the right.

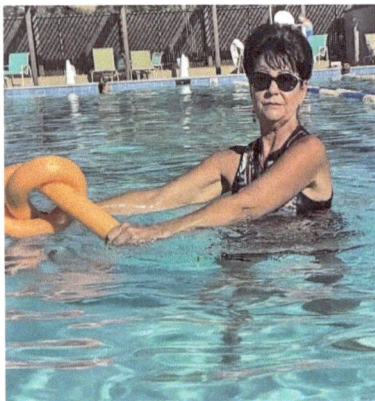

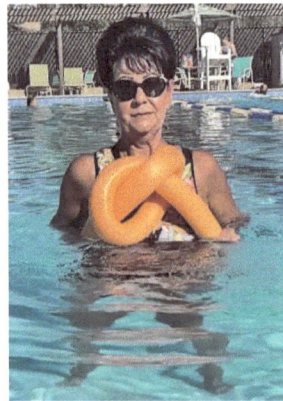

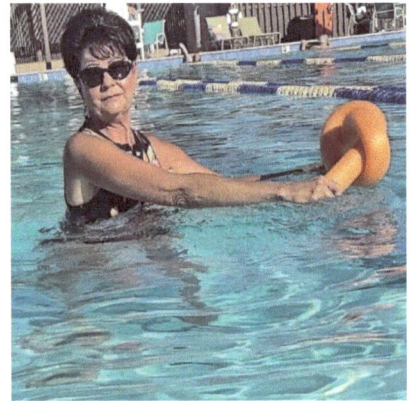

Repeat 20 to 25 times. Each side, left/right is counted as one push/pull.

ACTION: Bringing the noodle into the chest engages the scapular retractors, shoulder extensors and elbow flexors. Pushing the pretzel to the left engages the left trunk rotators, left hip internal rotators, right hip external rotators, shoulder flexors, and elbow extensors. Pushing the noodle to the right engages the same muscles on the opposite side of the body.

Pretzel with "Ears Up"

Helps strengthen arm, shoulder, and upper torso muscles. Improves body stability.

The noodle remains in a knotted position. Maintain a capital letter A stance with legs, and feet facing forward. Place the noodle with the ends up ("ears up") in the right hand, straighten arm out to the right side on the water's surface. The right straight arm pulls/pushes the pretzel noodle down and up about 6 to 8 inches from the water's surface 12 times.

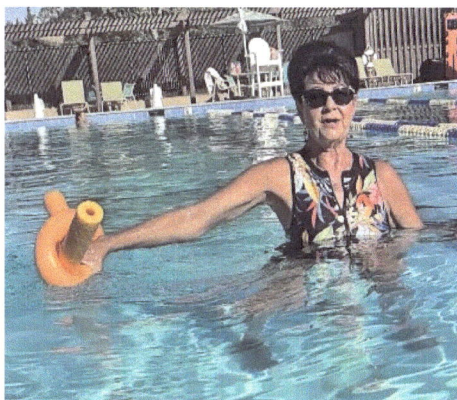
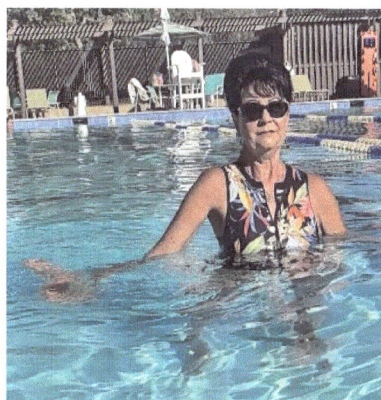

Then, place pretzel noodle in your left hand ("ears up") with the straight arm out to the left side. The left straight arm pulls/pushes the pretzel noodle down and up about 6 to 8 inches from the water's surface. Repeat 12 times.

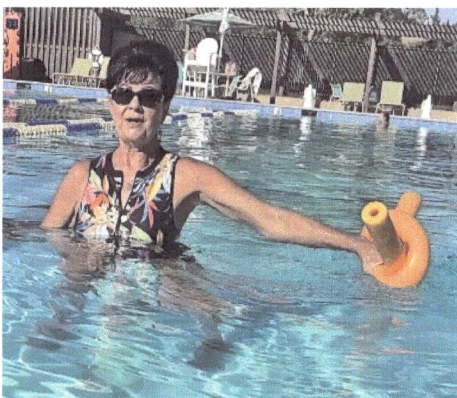
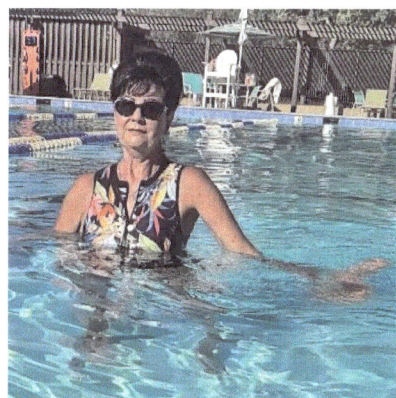

ACTION: Holding the arm out to the side and grabbing the noodle engages the shoulder abductors, elbow extensors, finger flexors and wrist stabilizers. Pulling the noodle down strengthens the shoulder adductors.

Allowing the arm to elevate is a release in the downward tension. The motion is an eccentric contraction of the shoulder adductors.

Pendulum Leg Kick

Helps flexibility of lower leg. Increases lower back strength and improves balance.

Stand in shallow water. For balance hold the noodle under the left forearm. With the right leg, flat foot, swing the right, straight leg forward and backward like the pendulum of a clock.

This forward/backward swinging of the straight leg is repeated 12 to 15 times. Repeat this swinging movement with the left straight leg, flat foot keeping the same pendulum movement.

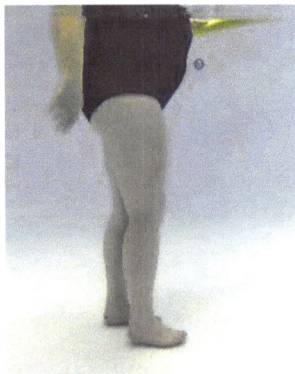

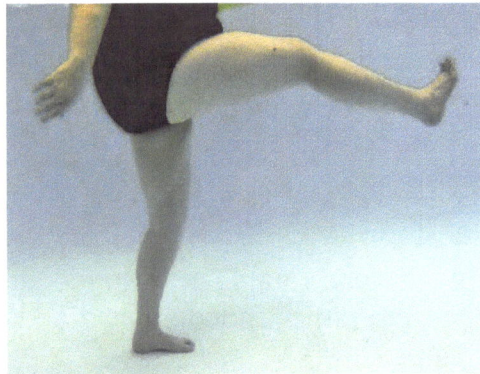

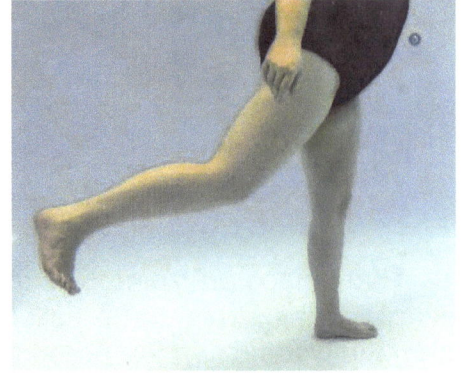

ACTION: Standing upright gives the body a strong anchoring point on the ground, but the trunk and pelvic stabilizers must still be active to decrease the amount of trunk sway in the water. This exercise is meant to target the lower extremities (legs). Kicking a straight leg out in front of the body requires activation of the hip flexors, knee extensors and ankle dorsiflexors. Bringing the leg back behind the body engages the hip extensors, knee extensors and ankle dorsiflexors. When kicking behind the body, one must continue to engage the abdominals to avoid leaning the entire body forwards.

Knee Side Swing and Kick to Water Surface

Helps balance and spinal stability. Strengthens knees and hips.

The noodle remains under the left forearm.

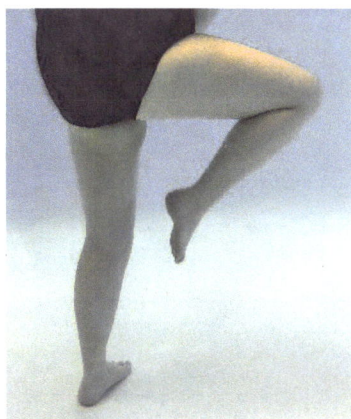

The knee is bent and kept at a ninety degree angle. It is swung to the right and back to the front of the torso for 12 to 15 times.

Keeping the right knee bent, move it to the side for the exercise below.

With the right knee out to the side, the right foot is raised to straighten the knee as close as possible to the water surface. The foot from the bent knee is raised and lowered 12 to 15 times.

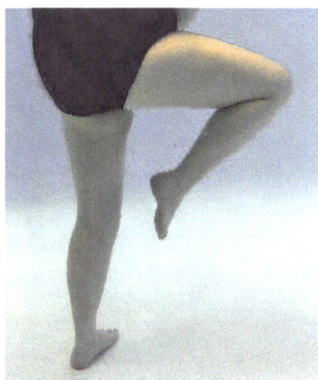

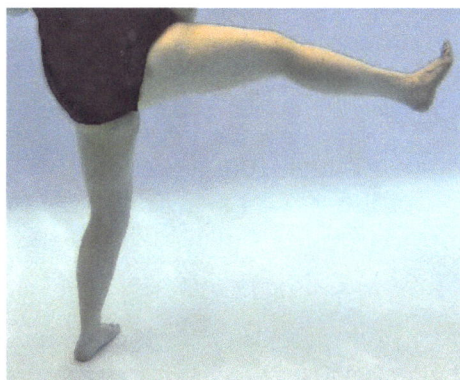

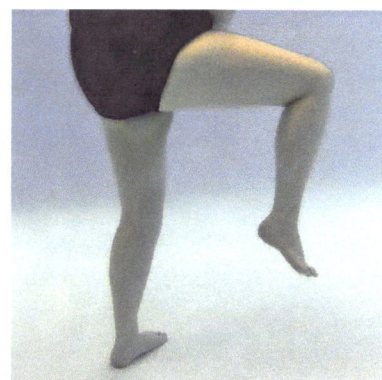

Repeat this exercise using the left leg.

ACTION: Lifting the knee engages the hip flexors while moving the knee to the side away from the left leg engages the hip abductors. The kicking and bending movement of the knee is achieved by alternating contractions of the knee extensors and knee flexors. The ankle dorsiflexors remain active throughout the exercise to keep the toe raised.

Standing on one leg further challenges the pelvic and trunk stabilizers as well.

Straight Leg Kick Across the Torso

Helps to stretch pelvic muscles and lower back. Improves balance and posture.

With the noodle remaining under the left forearm and the right leg turned to the side, the knee is straightened and brought as close to the water's surface as possible.

The straight, outstretched leg, with a flat foot is drawn from the side across the torso as far as possible.

This straight legged kick across the torso is repeated 12 to 15 times.

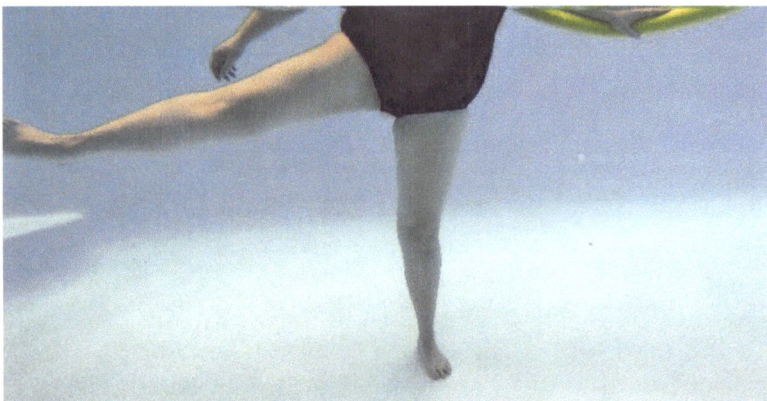

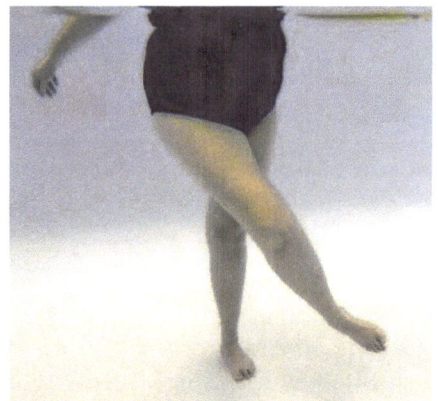

Repeat the exercise using the left leg.

ACTION: Standing on one leg will challenge the pelvic and trunk stabilizers to maintain balance and keep an upright posture.

Kicking the leg out to the side primarily engages the hip abductors and hip external rotators with a holding contraction of the knee extensors and ankle dorsiflexors. The inward swing crossing the body is performed by the hip adductors along with the same stabilizing muscles used in the outward swing.

Windshield Wiper

Helps stretch and strengthen small lower back muscles near the spine. Improves balance, coordination, and posture.

NOTE: Avoid this exercise if you have had any type of hip replacement.

With the noodle remaining under the left forearm, the right leg is kept straight and out to the side of the torso.

The straight right leg is pulled downward toward the left leg. Then, the right leg with a flat foot is pulled and pushed with the right heel and ankle in front of the left leg, with small, rapid movements like a windshield wiper.

Repeat this rapid foot movement 30 times. Then brings the leg downward and places both feet on the bottom of the pool.

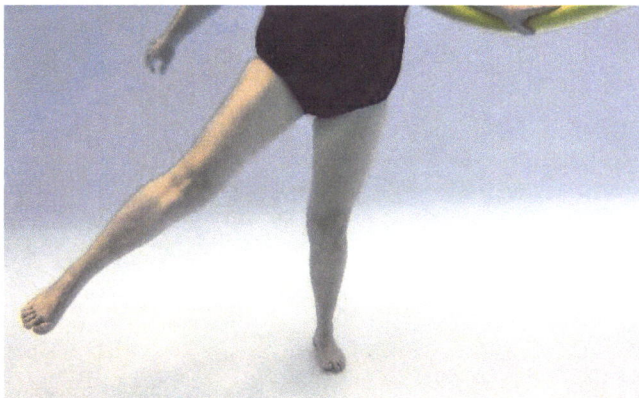

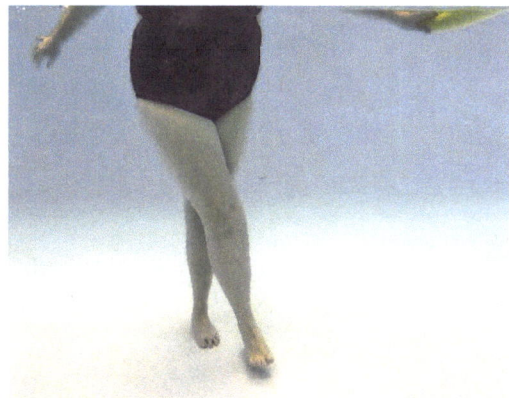

Repeat the exercise using the left leg.

ACTION: The rapid alternating short arc movement of one foot in front of the other is a motion that starts at the pelvis. The movement requires an isometric, stabilizing contraction of the Latissimus Dorsi and Quadratus Lumborum muscles to keep the pelvis stable and preventing it from moving up and down. Rapid, alternating concentric contractions recruit the hip adductors and abductors.

Due to the quick movements involved, sustaining a strong abdominal contraction is required to maintain trunk stability during this exercise.

Ballerina

Helps to stretch lateral (side) abdominal and shoulder muscles.

The noodle remains under the left forearm and both feet stay on the pool floor. The feet are shoulder distance apart in a comfortable stance. Raise the right arm bringing it over the head. The elbow is bent as the arm comes across the head and over the torso toward the left side of the body. The arm moves back to the stretched-out position without touching the water. This "ballerina" movement is repeated 12 to 15 times. Repeat this same exercise using the left arm.

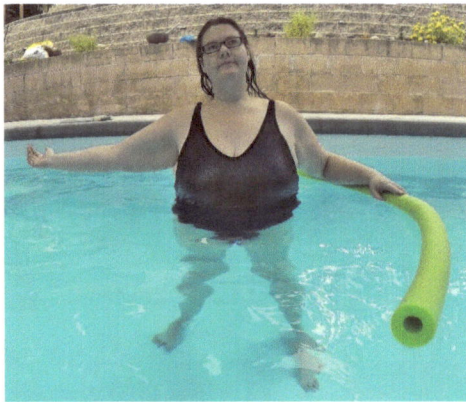

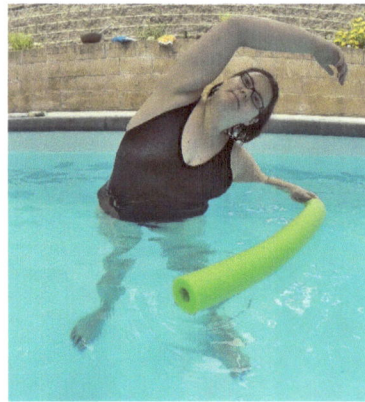

ACTION: Reaching up and over the head engages the shoulder abductors and external rotators. Leaning the torso to the side engages the lateral abdominals on the side you're leaning towards and stretches the other. Returning to an upright position engages the opposite side of the body.

Walking #1
(Alternating legs)

Helps stretch lower back and pelvic muscles. Strengthens legs. Improves balance.

Place the noodle in front of the torso for balance. Facing forward, pull one leg up as if to kick. The flat foot is then pushed behind as the leg straightens. The straightened leg is pulled backwards to the pool floor as the other leg performs the same motion. Walking backwards completely across the pool is highly recommended. Turn around and walk backwards to complete a second circuit.

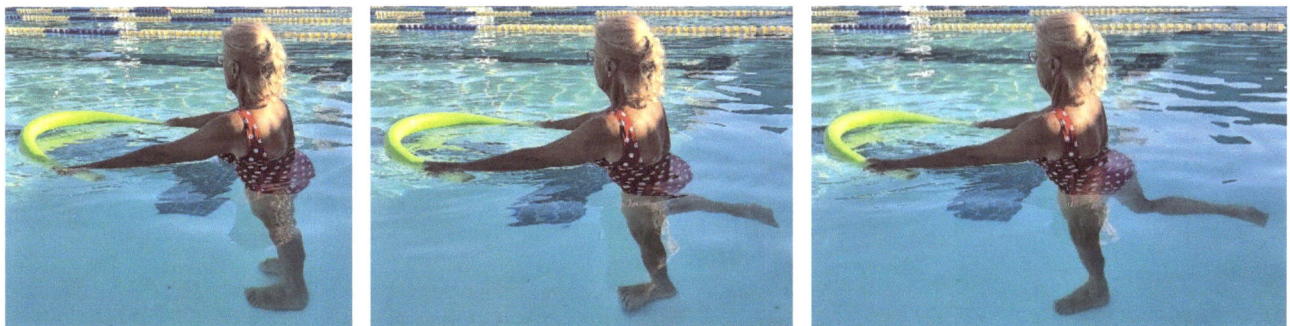

ACTION: Pulling one leg up to kick the rear end is an action of the knee flexors. Pushing the flat foot behind the body then engages the hip extensors, knee extensors and ankle dorsiflexors. Bringing the straight leg back down to the ground activates the hip flexors until the toe touches the ground. Pulling the body backwards with that leg as the other one lifts requires a strong contraction of the hip flexors on the standing leg.

When pushing the leg back to take a step, it is important to think about squeezing the buttock muscles and abdominals. Some tend to use their back muscles to move their leg, but this could lead to overuse so it is important to use the buttock muscles instead.

111

Walking #2
(Alternating legs, like a modified can-can)

Helps improve balance and coordination. Strengthens knees, hips, and legs.

Face one side of the pool. Place noodle in front of the torso for balance.

Pulled knee upwards from the pool floor. Straighten leg in front of the torso and then pull it back to the pool floor as the other leg performs the same motion. The person walks forward across the pool, turns around and walks back across the pool a second time.

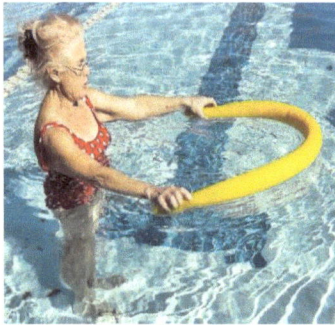

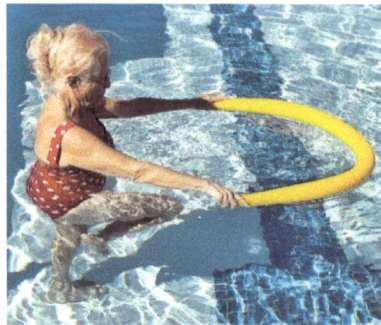

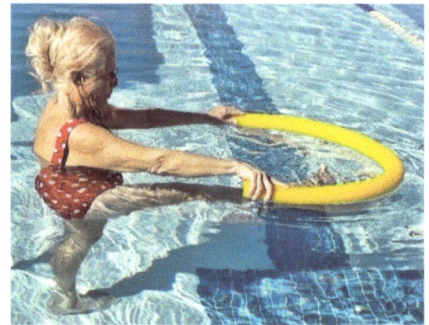

ACTION: The noodle is maintained in front of the torso by the shoulder and arms. The buoyancy of the noodle allows muscular effort of the shoulder and arms to aid in balance during the lower extremity exercise. The lower extremity muscle effort to elevate the thighs, straighten the knee, and advance the leg forward and downward to a flat foot is achieved by the hip flexors, knee extensors and ankle dorsiflexors. The knee and hip are extended behind the body as the opposite side of the body begins to lift and advance the leg.

It is important to maintain contraction of abdominal muscles, spinal muscles, and pelvic muscles to keep an erect posture throughout the exercise and help maintain balance.

Walking #3

Helps strengthen knees, ankles, and pelvic muscles. Increases lower body flexibility.

Face the side of the pool. Toes are placed pointing outwards. Walk across the shallow end of the pool with toes pointing outward (Charlie Chaplin). Then, turn around and faces the opposite side of the pool.

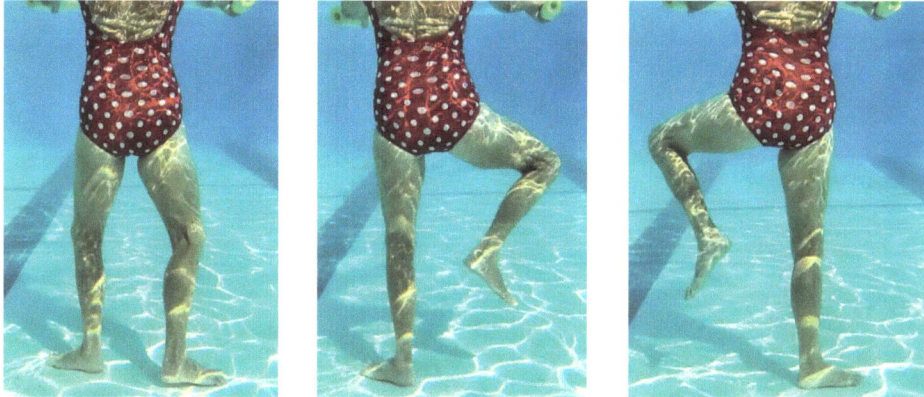

ACTION: The "Charlie Chaplin" walk is a high-step walk. The hip externally rotates and flexes to raise the thigh. External rotation of the thigh engages the deep external rotators of the hip and raising the thigh engages the hip flexors. Due to the new orientation of the legs (toes out), advancing the leg forward engages the hip adductors located on the inner aspect of the thigh. Bringing the leg back down to the pool floor utilizes the hip extensors, knee extensors and ankle stabilizers.

Walking #4

Turn toes inward. Walk across the pool with toes pointing inward (pigeon-toed). Turn once again to face the opposite side of the pool.

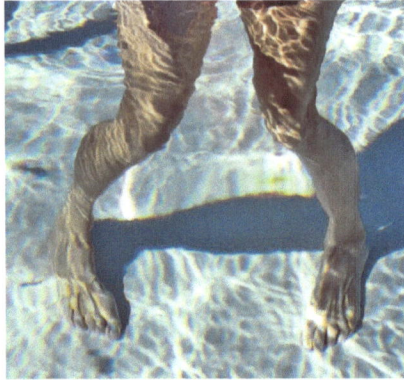

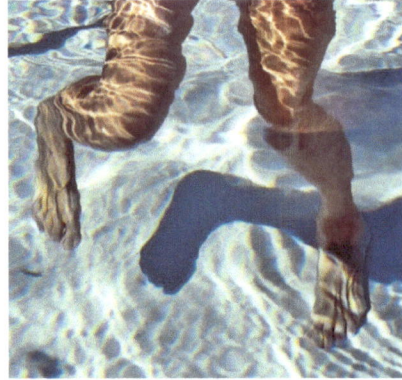

ACTION: Walking "pigeon toed" is also a high step walk. Achieving the position of the toes is primarily done with the hip internal rotators. Lifting the thigh activates the hip flexors and advancing the legs involves more of the hip abductors and flexors due to the orientation of the toes. Be careful not to bring your toes too far into the pigeon-toed stance if you have any history of knee pain as this can cause tension and excess pressure at the knees.

Walking #5

Helps to strength ankles and Achilles' tendons. Improves balance, posture and spinal alignment.

Bring knees and ankle close together and raise up on the toes. Walk across the pool on tiptoes, turning around and then walk across on the heel of the foot.

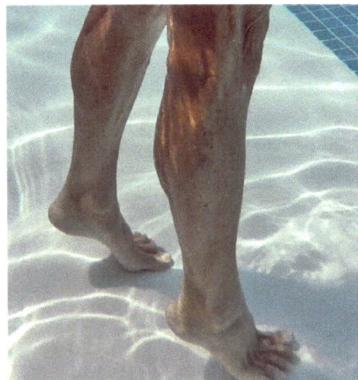

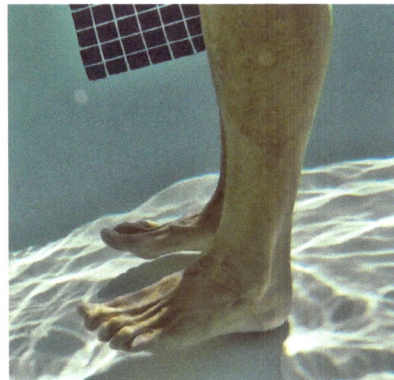

ACTION: Raising up on the toes is an action of the ankle plantar flexors. Walking across the pool on tip toes requires full body control as you don't achieve the usual biomechanical advantages from ankle position that assist with walking. To lift the thigh and advance the leg, the hip flexors and knee extensors must engaged. Once the foot hits the ground, the hip extensors kick in to help pull the torso over the leg and advance the body forward.

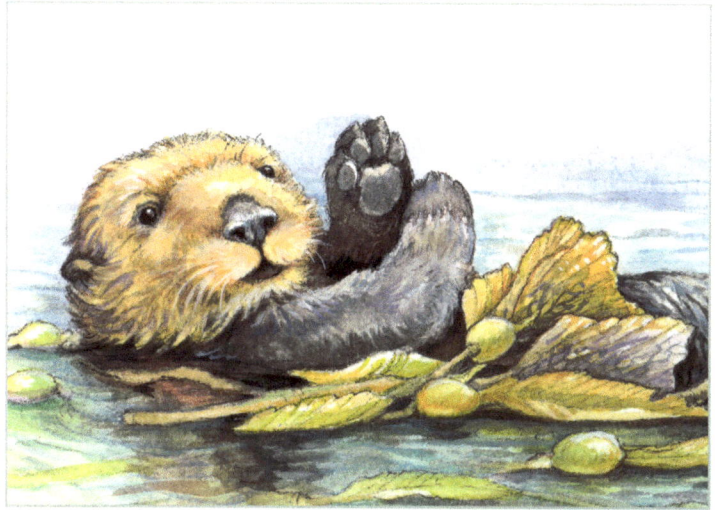

COOL DOWN

> *"Water aerobics classes have helped my stiff and painful joints. I have been able to accomplish my goal of losing weight and increasing my fitness. I have truly enjoyed the classes."*
> – Carol W.

Pre-Exercise Information for Cool Down

A cool down for water aerobics is essential. At the end of each workout a 10-15 minute session should involve slow movement and stretching. Without a cool down light headedness and dizziness can occur.

Water aerobics elevates the heart rate increasing blood flow to the lower extremities. Adrenaline is pumping through the body. Rapid breathing gives more oxygen to the body, and body temperature increases. Muscles are more relaxed and flexible.

Benefits of a cool down bring the body back to normalcy, gradually cooling the body temperature.

The chances of muscle cramping becomes less; injuries are reduced; and breathing becomes more normal. Relaxed muscles increase range of motion in the joints. The brain begins to release endorphins, Dopamine and serotonin. Motivation increases and feelings of relaxation and rejuvenation happen.

Performing gentle, cool down movements at the end of a workout will decrease blood pooling in the veins, arteries, and capillaries of the lower extremities. When muscles contract and relax, they form a type of pump that helps push blood back up to the heart. With a cool down, blood is allowed to be redistributed throughout the body. Cooling down reduces and delays onset muscle soreness and lessens the possibility of pain.

Hula Hoop

Helps increase flexibility of pelvic area and waist. Improves lower back movement.

Stand in shallow water. Place legs with feet about shoulder distance apart.

Rotate pelvis and hips to the right in a small circle approximately 15 to 20 times. Then, change the direction of the rotation. Rotate pelvis and hips to the left in a small circle approximately 15 to 20 times.

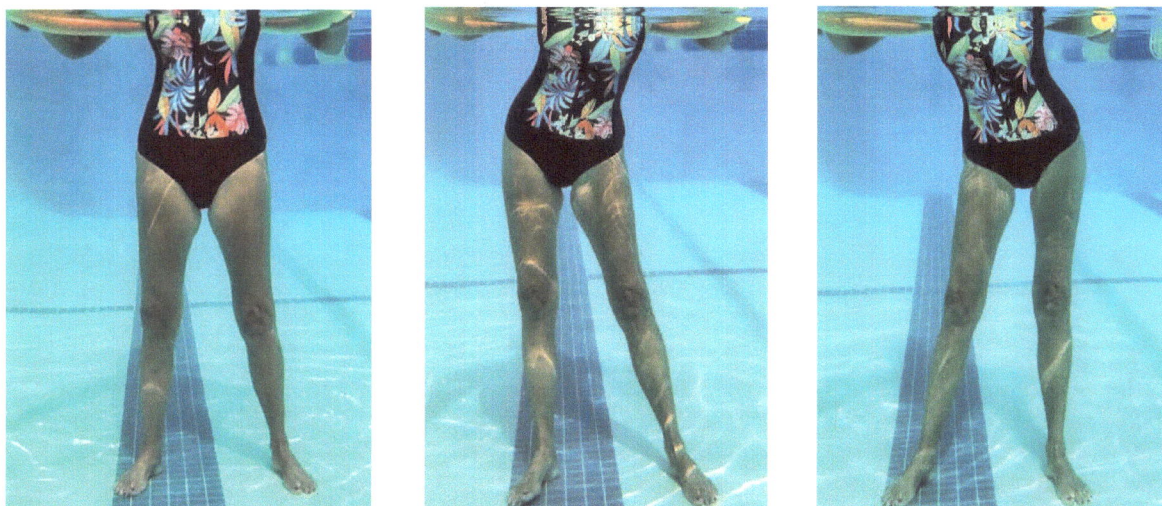

ACTION: Rotation is an action of the pelvis rotating about the head of the femur on the hip joint. The rotation of the pelvis around the hip joint is a sequence of muscles activating one after another all around the body. Pushing the hip out to the right engages the right hip adductors, left hip abductors, and left trunk side bending muscles. Pushing the pelvis forward is relative engagement of the hip extensors and back extensors. Pushing the hips to the left engages the left hip adductors, right hip abductors and right trunk side bending muscles. Finally, pushing the pelvis backwards engages the hip and trunk flexors. These muscle groups all take turns activating then releasing their tension to allow the other muscle groups to move the pelvis in a smooth circle.

Crab Walk

Helps strengthen and stretch ankles and feet. Increases lower leg flexibility.

NOTE: Avoid the exercise if you've had an anterior hip replacement.

Stand in shallow water with feet shoulder distance apart, forming a capital letter A.

Turn the toes outward and begin walking. One heel (right foot) and one set of toes (left foot) moving toward the right. Repeat alternating heel/toes movement about 8 times before changing direction and moving toward the left.

The alternating heel/toes movement is repeated another 8 times in the opposite direction. Then, the complete exercise is repeated right to left movement alternating heels and toes 12-15 times.

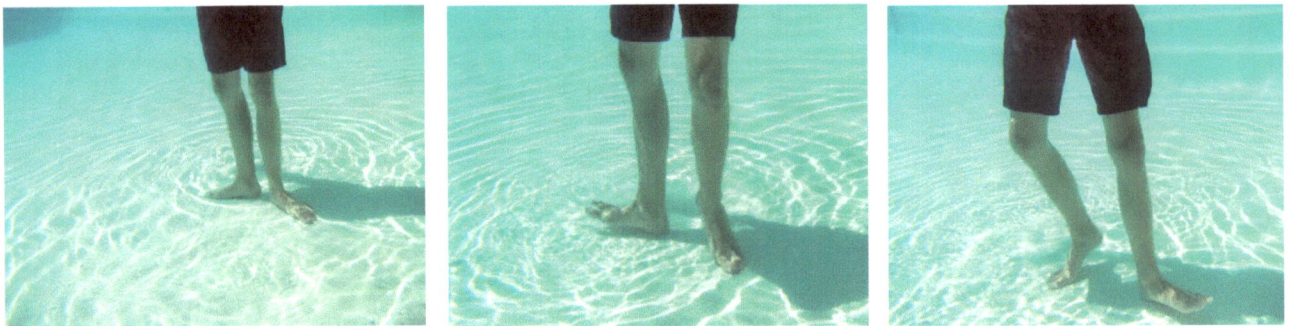

ACTION: The crab walk begins in the same position like a Charlie Chaplin walk with the toes pointed out. This position is achieved by the hip external rotators. Instead of walking forwards, the crab walk is performed to the side. When walking to the right, the right hip abductors and flexors help pull the leg to the side and the knee extensors must stabilize the leg position so the knee does not bend as it pushes through the water. Bringing the left leg back into midline engages the left hip adductors and extensors. The right hip adductors, knee flexors and ankle plantar flexors may assist with this action as well.

The abdominals must be strong to help isolate the movement to the lower extremities and avoid having the trunk move back and forth as you walk from side to side.

Squats — Toes Out and Toes Forward

Helps increase hip flexibility and spinal alignment. Strengthens ankles, knees, and hips. Stretches lower back.

In shallow water, stand with feet shoulder distance apart, like a capital letter A. Point toes outward from the stance.

Squat, bending knees to an approximate 90-degree angle and returns to an upright position. Repeat downward/upward movement 12 to 15 times.

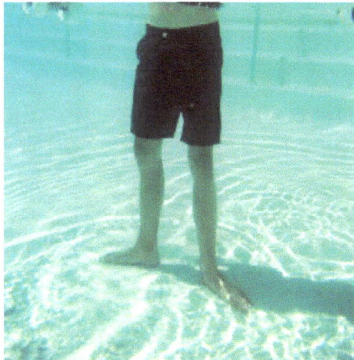

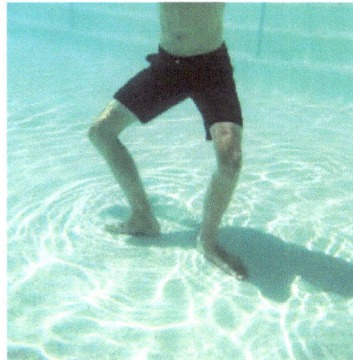

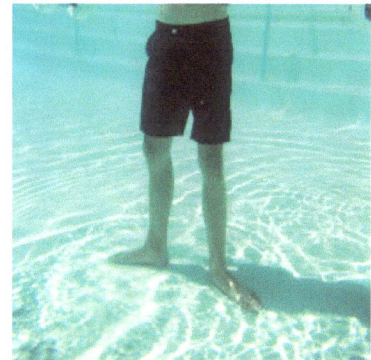

The same downward/upward squatting movement is repeated 12 to 15 times with the toes now pointing forward.

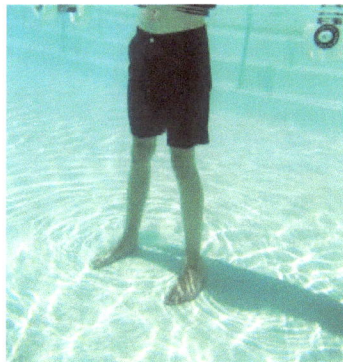

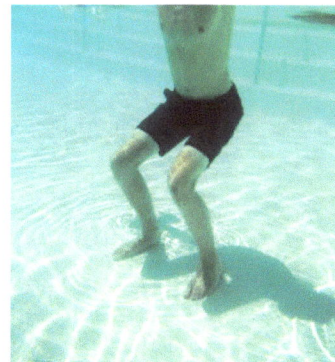

ACTION: Lowering the body into the squat involves an eccentric contraction of the hip extensors, knee extensors and ankle plantar flexors. Pushing the body back up involves a concentric contraction of these same muscles. Turning the toes out activates the hip external rotators and further challenges the hip adductors in the raising and lowering of the body.

Knee Pull Up
(With lower leg rotation and ankle flexes)

Helps posture and balance. Strengthens pelvic area. Increases knee and ankle flexibility.

Plant feet are firmly upon the pool floor, shoulder distance apart. Hold weights with bent elbows upon the water's surface so that the elbows are even with the shoulders. This position will help maintain balance. The left knee, foot, and ankle are elevated, and pulled upward to become even with the hip.

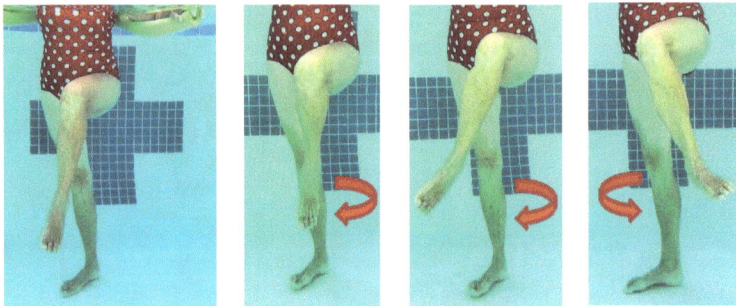

The lower leg, from the knee down, is rotated inward 12 times in a small circular motion. Change direction and lower leg outward 12 times.

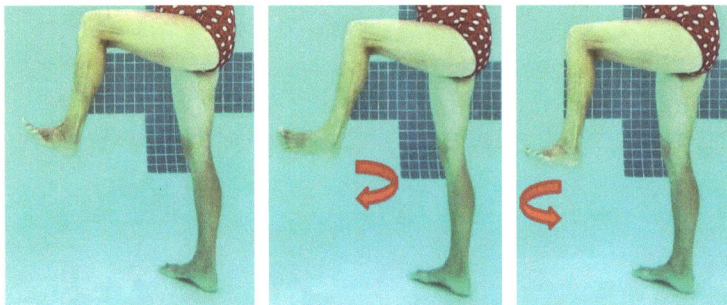

The upward leg position is kept in place and the foot is flexed downward/upward (wave good-bye to the pool floor) 12 times. At the completion of the ankle flexes, the foot is kept flat. The big toe is rotated in small circles inward/outward 12 times keeping the flat foot in front of the knee.

Repeat this exercise with the right leg.

ACTION: In this exercise, the body is anchored by the foot firmly on the pool floor and by the weights in the hands. Lifting the right thigh is easy because the left leg is firmly anchored in a single leg stance. This allows the pelvis to have stability for the hip muscles. Holding the weights offers stability to the shoulders, which in turn give stability to the abdominal and spinal muscles. These muscles help to contract and hold the torso erect on the pelvis. All that has been described has been a contraction of a muscle whose distal attachments have been anchored by the foot planted on the pool floor and weights in the hands. The lower extremity muscles contract and form this stable, anchored proximal attachment. Lifting the hip engages the hip flexors. The foot is rotated inward by the hip external rotators and outward by the internal rotators. Although this seems counterintuitive, when the foot is rotated outward, the front of the hip is being turned inwards, thus the internal rotation at the hip. To visualize this, if you make a fist with the thumb pointed upward, place the fist on the thigh just proximal to the knee. When you push the foot out, your thumb will point in. And when you bring your foot in, the thumb will point out. The right hip extension is an action of putting the foot on the pool floor engaging the Gluteus Maximus. The knee extension engages the Quadriceps muscle group. The right foot "waves goodbye" and engages the ankle dorsiflexors and plantar flexors.

Knee Pulls

Encourages Stretch of the Sciatic Nerve and Piriformis Muscle.

Helps balance, spinal alignment, and posture. Stretches lower back and pelvic area.

As in the previous exercise, the feet are firmly planted upon the pool floor shoulder distance apart. The weights are held with flexed elbows on the water's surface and slightly in front of the torso.

The right knee is elevated to touch the left elbow or wrist; then, the left knee is elevated to touch the right elbow or wrist.

This alternating movement is repeated approximately 25-26 times so that each elbow/wrist is alternately tapped by the opposite knee.

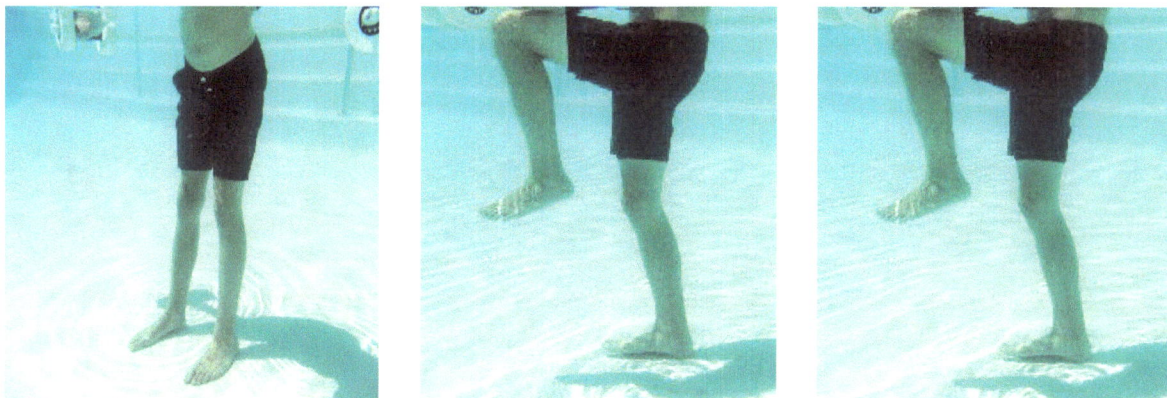

ACTION: In this exercise, the body is anchored by the foot firmly on the pool floor and by the weights in the hands.

Lifting the knee up and across the body engages the hip flexors, hip adductors, hip internal rotators and trunk rotators. Bringing the left knee to the right elbow or wrist involves left trunk rotation. This engages the left internal obliques and right external obliques, thus strengthening muscles on both sides of the body. Bringing the foot back down to the pool floor engages the hip extensors, knee extensors and hip external rotators.

Straight Leg Swings with a Circle

Helps strengthen hip and pelvic area. Stretches lower body muscles.

Stand in shallow water with legs held together. The right leg with a flat foot is pulled to the side of the torso.

Leading with the ankle and heel, pull the right leg across the torso and form a large circle in front of the torso bringing the right leg as close to the water's surface as possible.

After the right leg makes a large circle with a flat foot, it is returned to the starting position beside the left foot. Then, the same movement is repeated with the left leg. Pull the left leg across the torso and makes a large circle in front of the torso bringing the left leg as close to the water's surface as possible. After the left leg makes a large circle with the flat foot, it is returned to the starting position. The legs are <u>alternating</u> this right and left movement for approximately 12 times.

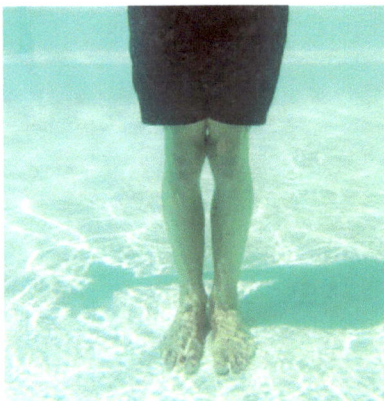

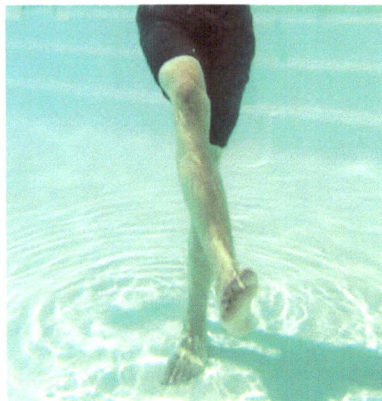

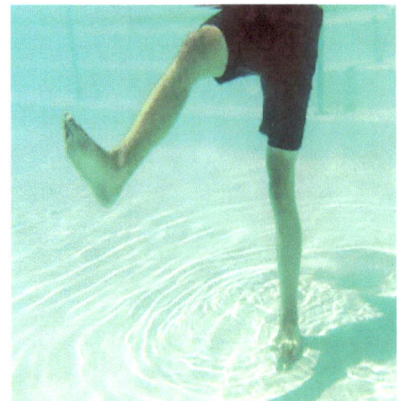

ACTION: Maintaining a flat foot throughout this exercise requires constant activation of the ankle dorsiflexors and keeping the leg straight the entire time is a constant contraction of the knee extensors. Pulling the straight leg across the torso engages the hip flexors and adductors. Keeping the leg elevated and bringing it back to the side of the body activates the hip flexors and hip abductors. Completing the circle engages the hip extensors and hip adductors.

The spinal and pelvic stabilizers must be active to keep the torso upright and stable while the legs move.

Straight-Legged Step Back

Helps stretch and strengthen lower back, foot and ankle. Increases body stability and spinal alignment.

Stand in shallow water with legs together.

The right flat foot is pulled backward from the torso approximately 5 inches keeping both feet flat. The right flat foot is placed upon the pool floor behind the torso and held flat upon the pool floor for about 30 seconds. Then, the right foot is brought back to the standing position.

The left flat foot is pulled backward from the torso approximately 5 inches keeping the foot flat. The left flat foot is placed upon the pool floor behind the torso and held flat upon the pool floor for about 30 seconds. Then, the left foot is brought back to the standing position.

Placing of right and left flat feet behind the torso with the foot held behind the torso. Hold first the right flat foot, and then hold the left flat foot behind is considered one time.

NOTE: Repeat this exercise 3 times only.

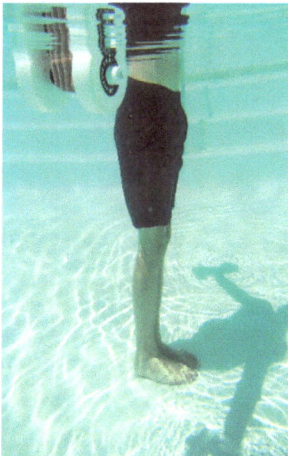

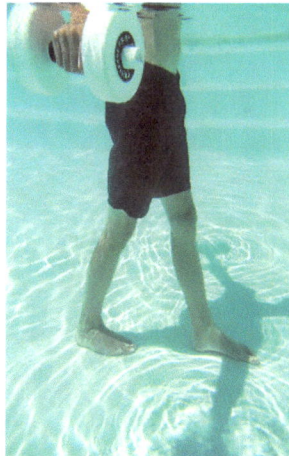

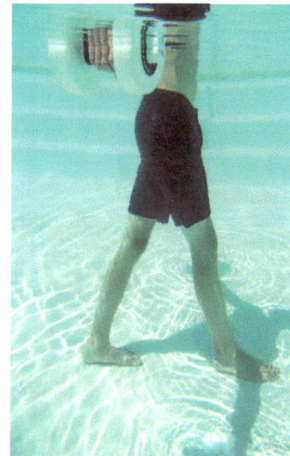

ACTION: This exercise engages the hip extensors to passively bring the ankle into dorsiflexion. Maintaining the foot flat stretches the heel cord, Achilles tendon and the two muscles attached to the tendon, the Gastrocnemius, and Soleus.

Toes and Heels

Helps strengthen Achilles tendon, ankles, and lower back. Stretches lower leg muscles. Improves spinal alignment and posture.

Stand with legs together in shallow water. The hand-held weights or noodle are held at a comfortable position near the shoulders to assist with balance.

Rise up on your toes and then rock backwards to the heels.

This rocking motion is repeated approximately 15 times.

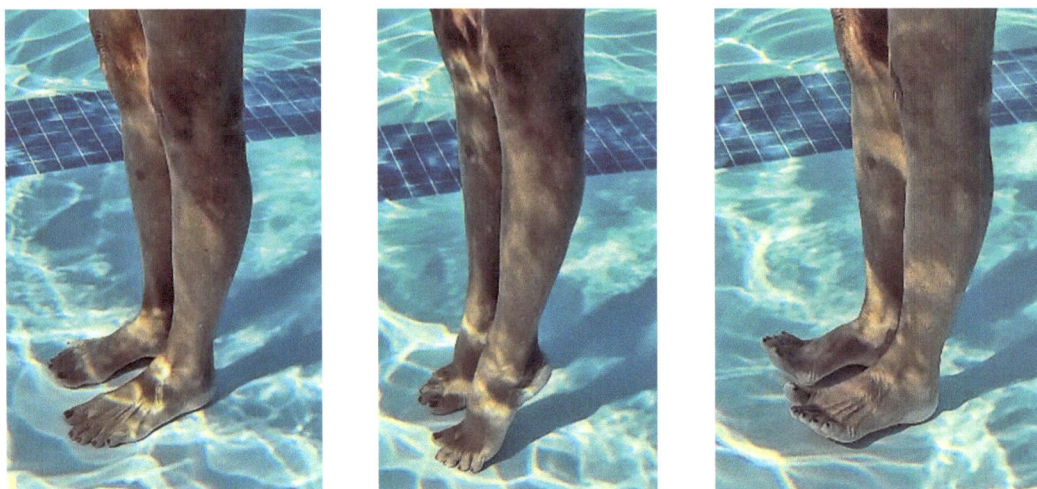

ACTION: Rising upward is a concentric contraction engaging the Gastrocnemius and Soleus muscles. The same muscles perform an eccentric contraction as they lower the heel to a flat foot position. Raising the toes and forefoot is a concentric contraction of the anterior tibialis at the ankle and the digitorum longus and hallucis longus at the toes.

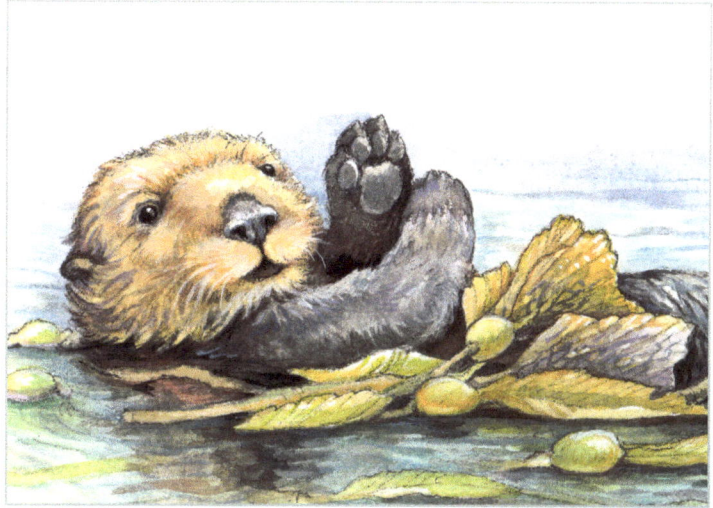

NECK

> "Just what little exercise I performed made me realize how out of shape I was. Water aerobics is energizing and a great cardio exercise too." – Michael L.

> "As a person with Parkinson's Disease, no balance and double knee replacements, water aerobics has really helped me to get my confidence back." – Linda H.

Neck Pre-Exercise Muscle Information

The neck helps provide overall functional strength. It is the "power behind the head." Neck exercises help relieve tension, reduce body pain, and increase flexibility. Neck exercises can decrease headaches and upper body pain. Stretching the scalene muscles (side of the neck) and the suboccipital muscles (lower back of the head and top of the neck) can increase blood flow and boost circulation. Posture is improved.

Keeping the neck flexible and conditioned can create and improve overall functional strength. A flexible, conditioned neck offers protection against injuries. It can keep the Eustachian tubes from clogging, which combats upper respiratory conditions. The Eustachian tube runs from the middle ear to the pharynx. Its function is to protect, aerate, and drain the middle ear and mastoid.

The photos in this section show detailed movements from my earlier book, *Water Wonder Works... A Guide To Therapeutic Exercises*.

The neck's main muscular support includes the deep neck flexors, suboccipitals, and cervical paraspinals. The deep neck flexors are located on the anterior aspect of the neck and include the longus colli, longus capitis, rectus capitis anterior and rectus capitis lateralis. These muscles collectively help retract the head to center it over the rest of the body. This movement centers the skull over the body's base of support, thereby minimizing the downward pull of gravity on one's posture. As our society evolves into desk-creatures, these muscles become even more important to combat the constant "forward head" posture that we fall into when staring at a screen or sitting at a desk.

The suboccipitals and cervical paraspinals are located on the posterior aspect of the neck. The suboccipitals are located at the base of the skull and the cervical paraspinal muscles are located on either side of the spine. These muscles help extend the neck and keep our eye line stable. With poor posture, the head begins to bend forward and down.

The upper trapezius muscles are a secondary, extrinsic support to the neck. These muscles, located on the top of the shoulders, are attached to the spine, shoulder blades, and skull. They are responsible for lifting the shoulders towards the ears and are very often shortened due to stress and poor movement patterns. Over activity of these muscles can lead to decreased neck mobility and headaches. Maintaining the mobility of these muscles is crucial to appropriate posture.

Freeway Exercise/Looking Back

Helps flexibility of the lateral (side) neck muscles.

Turn head slowly, first to the right and then slowly to the left, while holding the head level as if looking forward. Repeat 3 times.

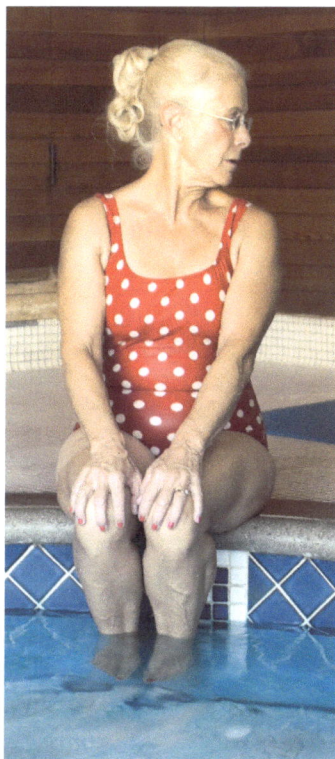

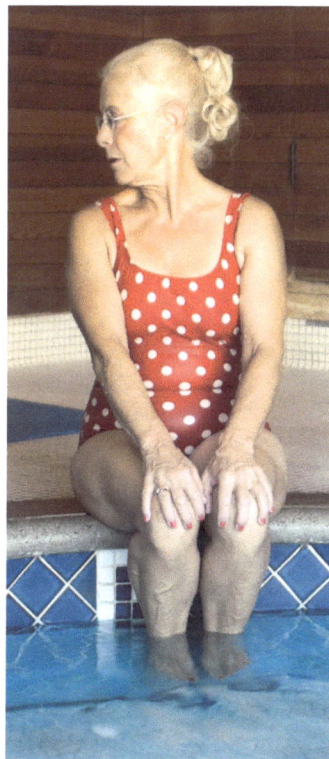

ACTION: Looking to the left activates the left-sided cervical parapinals and suboccipitals as well as the right-sided sternocleidomastoid and scalene muscles. Looking to the left also stretches the same muscles on the opposite sides of the neck. For example, if the left-sided cervical paraspinals are engaged to turn the head to the left, the right-sided cervical paraspinals will be stretched as the head turns.

Pendulum Neck Stretch

Helps flexibility of the back and Lateral (side) neck muscles.

Turn head slowly toward the left shoulder, keeping it upward and above the shoulder. Then, lower chin toward the left shoulder and slowly move to the right shoulder.

The chin moves and traces a slight curve across the collar bones. The head is brought slightly upward looking toward the right and above the shoulder.

The chin is brought slowly down toward the chest and slowly back to the left shoulder, making the same curve in the opposite direction. Complete 3 to 4 times, making each left to right and back one repetition.

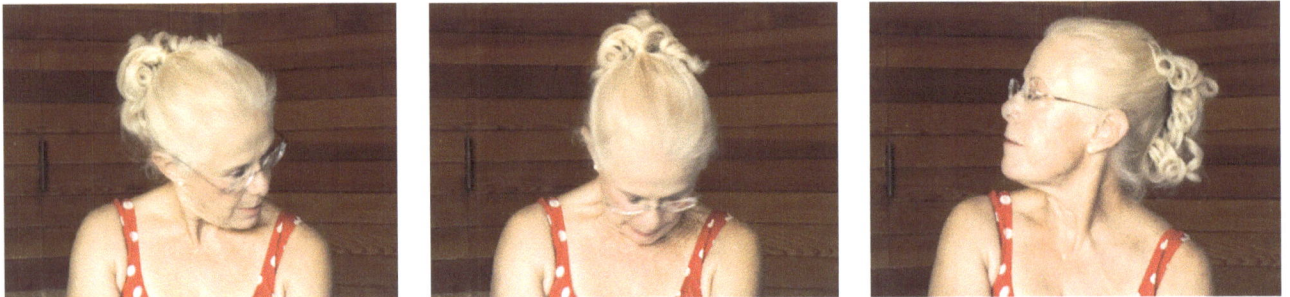

ACTION: This exercise is made up of many different motions at the neck. First, turning the head slowly to look at the left shoulder is called left rotation. This engages the left sided cervical paraspinals and suboccipitals as well as the right-sided sternocleidomastoid and scalenes. From here, lowering the chin to the shoulder is cervical flexion with rotation and engages the deep neck flexors on top of all the other aforementioned muscles. Bringing the chin to the right shoulder is called right rotation with flexion and the right-sided cervical paraspinals, and suboccipitals, and left-sided sternocleidomastoid and scalenes are activated with the deep neck flexors. Finally, bringing the head slightly upward to look above the right shoulder engages the cervical extensors: splenius capitis, splenius cervicis, cervical paraspinals, and the suboccipitals. Bringing the head back to the other side engages all the muscles in the reverse order.

Whenever you activate one muscle, you also stretch it's opposite (antagonist). For example, if you engage the left rotators, this stretches the right rotators. Similarly, whenever you activate the cervical flexors, the cervical extensors are stretched. In an exercise using all the muscles in sequence, you are also getting a stretch of the opposite (antagonist) muscles.

Nods

Helps flexibility of front and back neck muscles. May slow formation of a double chin. Look straight ahead. Nod up and down from the chest up.

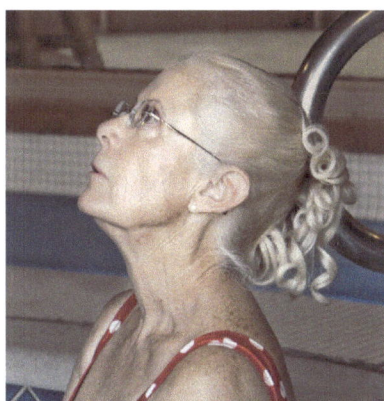

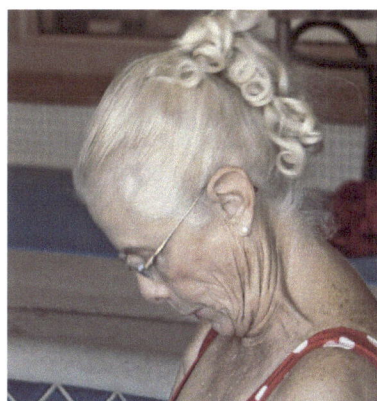

After the third repetition, the chin remains on the chest and is turned no more than 1 inch to first the left and then the right.

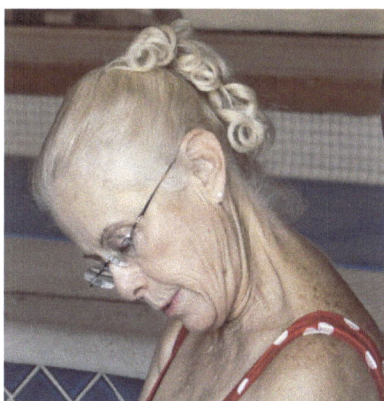

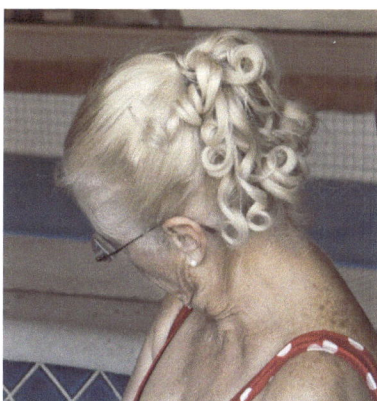

ACTION: Nodding the chin up and down engages and stretches the cervical flexors and extensors in an alternating pattern. Looking up will engage the cervical paraspinals and suboccipitals while stretching the deep neck flexors. Looking down will do the opposite.

Rotating the head while looking down engages the deep neck flexors and cervical rotators and provides a stretch to the posterior neck muscles and upper back.

Turtle Pull

Helps parallel head position as it stretches front, back and chin muscles.

The person is looking straight ahead. The arms are pulled back parallel to the torso. The hands are placed at mid-thigh position or behind the buttocks, so that the shoulders feel as if the hands are in the back pocket of a pair of jeans.

The chin is pulled inward toward the spine, and then pushed outward to the original position. "Push a drawer into the cupboard; pull the drawer out of the cupboard."

After the third repetition, the chin remains pulled back to the spine and is turned no more than 1 inch from left to right.

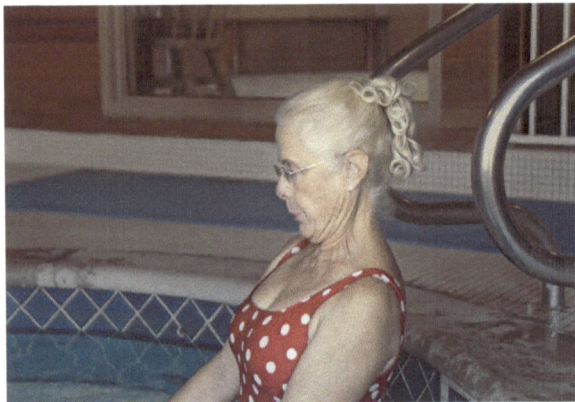

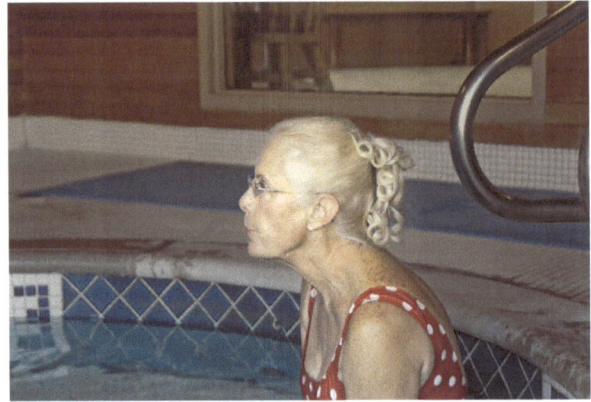

ACTION: The deep neck flexors bring the head back while keeping the chin stable. There is a difference between this movement and looking down towards the floor. When looking all the way down, the lower cervical flexors are active and this rotates the head down. When pulling the head back, the upper cervical flexors are active, shifting the entire head back without rotating it up or down.

As we work more at desks and drive further commutes, our resting posture becomes closer to the picture on the right, for example, slumped forward. This puts pressure on our spines and loads the vertebrae and muscles in abnormal ways. Pulling the head back strengthens the deep neck flexors, which will help maintain good posture throughout the day.

Muscle Glossary

Upper Extremity Muscle Groups:

- **Shoulder flexors:** Anterior deltoid, Coracobrachialis, Biceps brachii, Pectoralis major
- **Shoulder extensors:** Posterior deltoid, Latissimus Dorsi, Triceps brachii (long head), Teres major
- **Shoulder internal rotators:** Anterior deltoid, Latissimus Dorsi, Subscapularis, Teres major, Pectoralis major
- **Shoulder external rotators:** Posterior deltoid, Infraspinatus, Teres minor
- **Shoulder abductors:** Middle deltoid, Supraspinatus, Anterior deltoid, Posterior deltoid
- **Shoulder adductors:** Pectoralis major, Latissimus Dorsi, Teres major, Coracobrachialis
- **Shoulder horizontal abductors:** Posterior deltoid, Latissimus Dorsi, Teres major and minor, Infraspinatus
- **Shoulder horizontal adductors:** Pectoralis major, Subscapularis, Coracobrachialis, Anterior deltoid
- **Scapular retractors:** Upper, Middle and Lower Trapezius, Rhomboid major and minor, Latissimus Dorsi
- **Scapular protractors:** Pectoralis major and minor, Serratus anterior
- **Elbow extensors:** Triceps brachii, Anconeus
- **Elbow flexors:** Biceps brachii, Brachialis, Brachioradialis
- **Forearm pronators:** Pronator teres, Pronator quadratus, Brachioradialis
- **Forearm supinators:** Supintor, Biceps brachii, Brachioradialis
- **Wrist flexors:** Flexor digitorum superficialis and profundus, Flexor carpi radialis, Flexor carpi ulnaris, Palmaris Longus
- **Wrist extensors:** Extensor carpi radialis longus and brevis, Extensor digitorum, Extensor carpi ulnaris
- **Wrist radial deviators:** Flexor carpi radialis, Extensor carpi radialus longus and brevis
- **Wrist ulnar deviators:** Flexor carpi ulnaris, Extensor carpi ulnaris

Muscle Glossary continued on following page

Lower Extremity Muscle Groups:

- **Hip flexors:** Psoas, Iliacus, Sartorius, Tensor Fascia Latae

- **Hip extensors:** Gluteus Maximus, Gluteus medius, Gluteus minimus, Piriformis

- **Hip internal rotators:** Adductor longus, brevis and magnus, Tensor Fascia Latae, Pectineus

- **Hip external rotators:** Gluteus Maximus, Gluteus Medius, Gluteus Minimus, Piriformis, Psoas, Iliacus, Sartorius

- **Hip abductors:** Gluteus Medius, Gluteus Minimus, Sartorius, Tensor Fascia Latae, Piriformis

- **Hip adductors:** Adductor longus, brevis and magnus, Gracilis

- **Knee flexors:** Biceps femoris, Semimembranosus, Semitendinosus, Popliteus, Gracilis

- **Knee extensors:** Rectus femoris, Vastus Lateralis, Vastus Medialis, Vastus Intermedius

- **Ankle plantarflexors:** Gastrocnemius, Soleus, Plantaris, Tibialis Posterior, Peroneus longus and brevis, Flexor Digitorum Longus, Flexor Hallucis Longus

- **Ankle dorsiflexors:** Tibialis Anterior, Extensor Digitorum Longus, Extensor Hallucis Longus, Pernoeus Tertius

Axial Muscle Groups:

- **Trunk flexion:** Rectus Abdominis, External and Internal Obliques

- **Trunk extension:** Thoracic and Lumbar Paraspinals, Multifidi, Quadratus Lumborum, Rotatores

- **Sidebend:** Internal and External Obliques, and Thoracic and Lumbar Paraspinals, Quadratus Lumborum, Multifidi

- **Rotation (to the left):** left Internal Obliques, right External Obliques, right Multifidi, and Thoracic and Lumbar Paraspinals

- **Rotation (to the right):** left Internal Obliques; left External Obliques, left Multifidi, and Thorasic and Lumbar Paraspinals

Major Muscle Groups - Front
(an artistic creation)

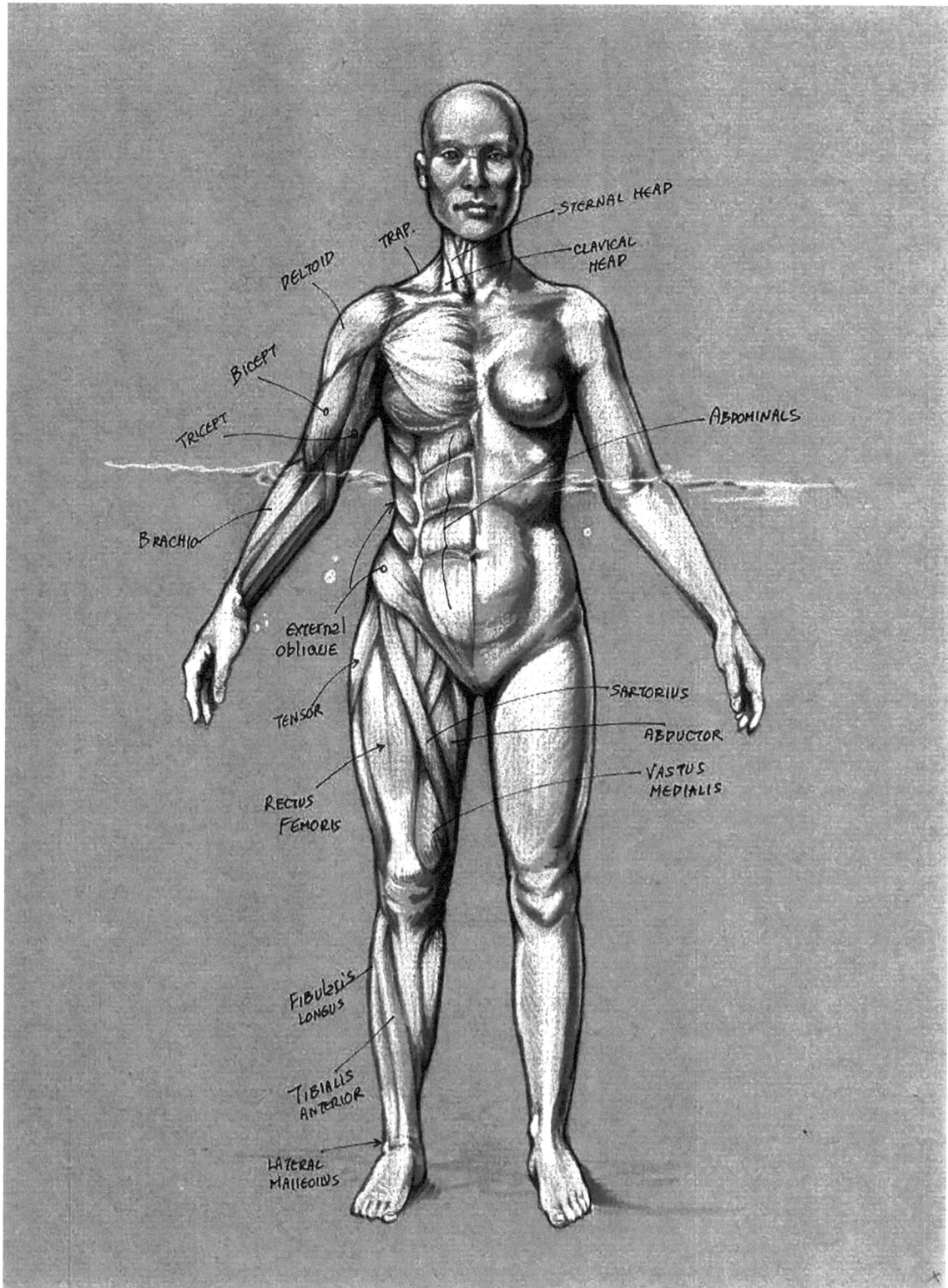

Major Muscle Groups - Back
(an artistic creation)

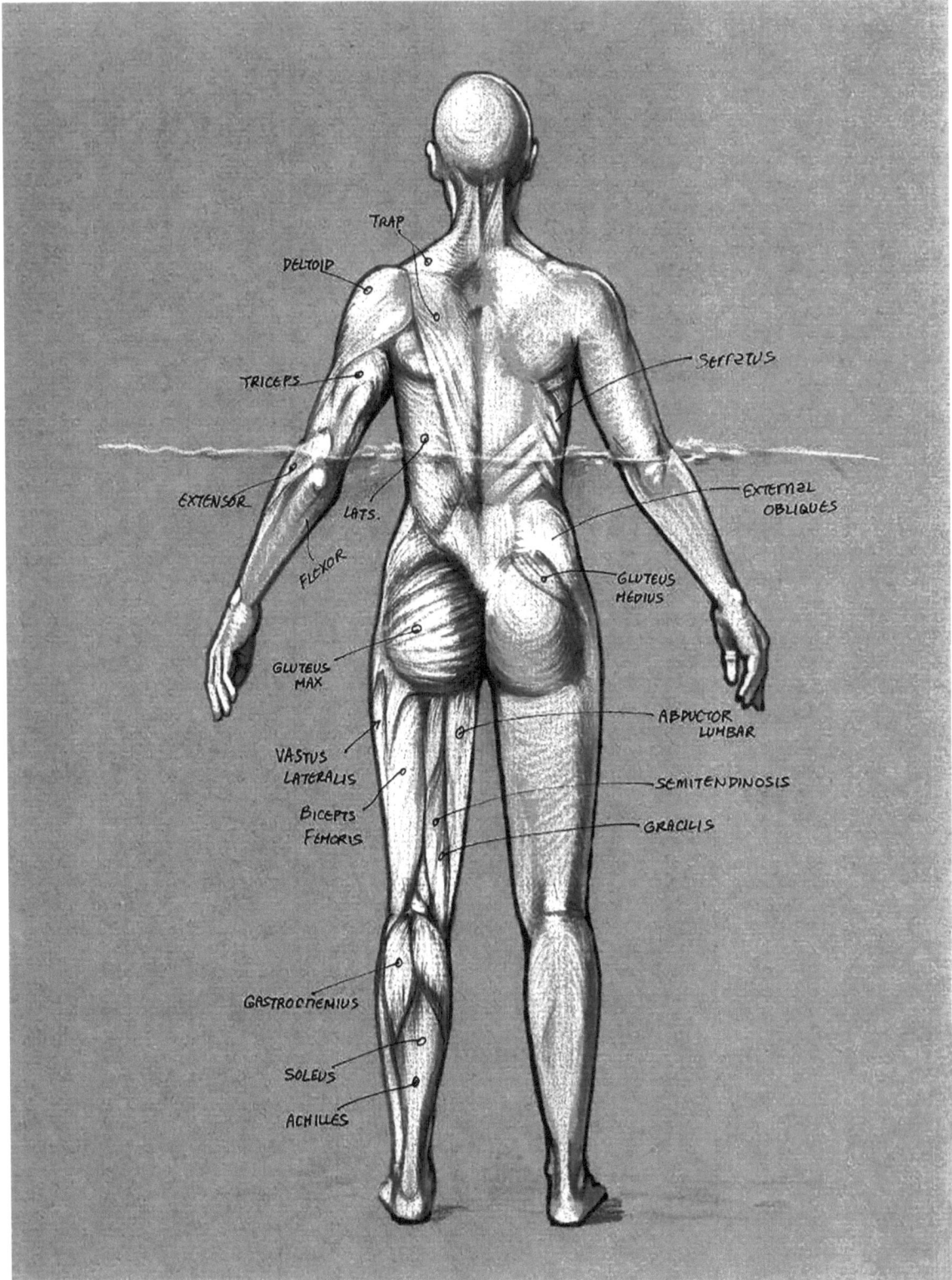

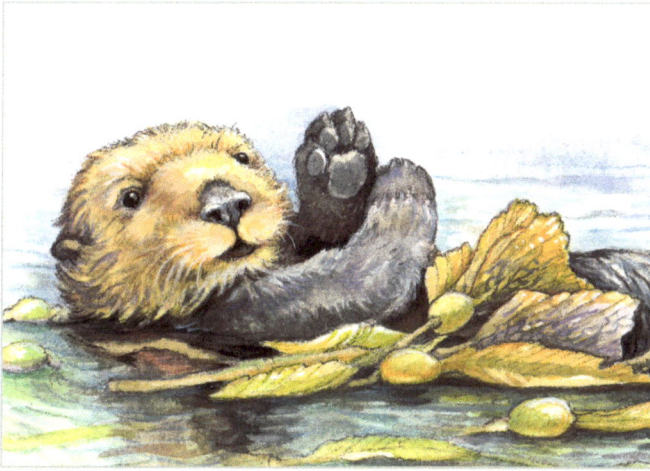

Love Notes

"Water Aerobics helps me with my autoimmune disease. With all my joints hurting, getting in the water to exercise is much easier for me. I also appreciate the emotional and social lift it always gives." – Debbie C.

"The exercises in water aerobics allow you to exercise without the fear of falling or hurting yourself. Three months after having a knee replacement, I took Marti's class with amazing results. I am more in balance and more fit." – Margaret P.

"I just had open heart surgery. Thanks to water aerobics I was in excellent shape. I am back in class now. The class has helped my recovery. Marti's class has helped me tremendously." – Kathleen M.

"After an accident at 18 years of age, I developed arthritis in both my knees and feet, and throughout my body. I also have asthma. Water aerobics was approved by my physicians. When I work in the water, I feel less pain. I have more flexibility. Water exercises have become very healing for me." – Valerie M.

"A few months ago, I was in an auto accident and suffered a whiplash. After three months of water aerobics my pain is less. I only need to take medication occasionally due to the strengthening from the water exercises." – Kristina W.

"Water aerobics is my life saver. After heart surgery, I have been able to feel and get my life back to a more normal state. I don't know what I would do without water aerobics." – Joan P.

Photo Credits

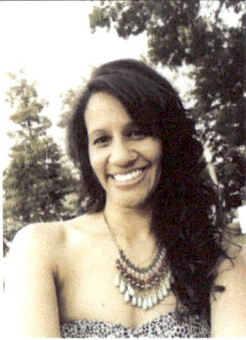
Kamillah S - Violinist |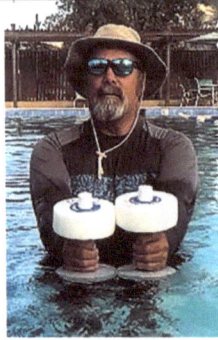
Mike W – Ret Businessman |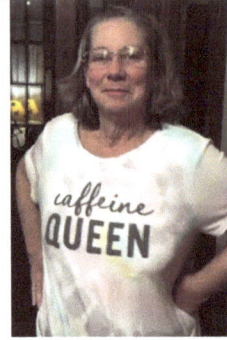
Donna M – USN Ret
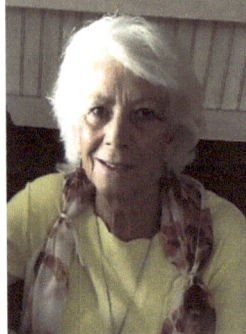
Wanda F – RN Ret |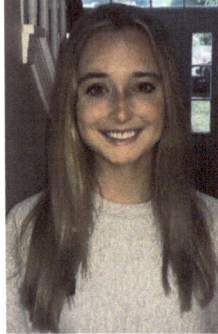
Carolina D - Student |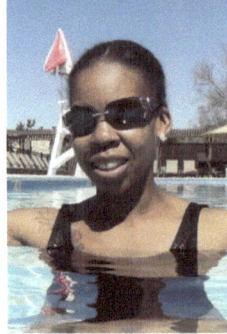
Courtney B – Culinary Artist
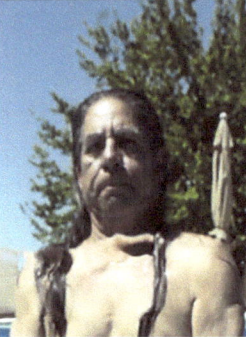
Mike L – Tribal Gourd Dancer |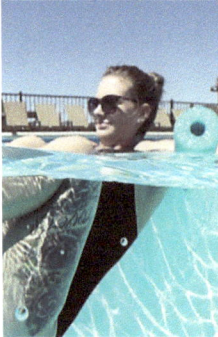
Olivia M – Culinary Artist |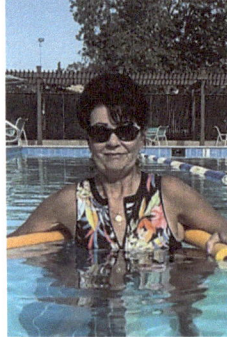
Joan B – Ret Exec Secretary
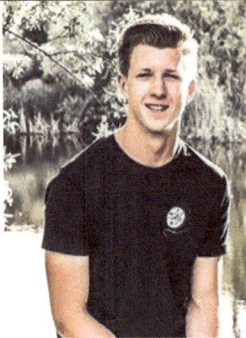
Dalton B – Lifeguard/Firefighter |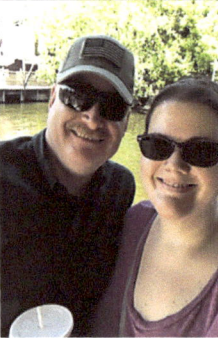
Rusty and Malissa W
Ret Military/Former EMT-P |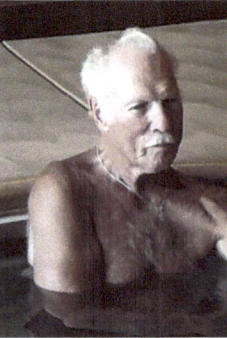
Jay S – Ret Police Officer

Bibliography

Biel, Andrew. <u>Trail Guide to the Body…How to locate muscles, bones and more.</u> Andrew Biel. Boulder,CO. printed by Consolidated Press. Seattle, WA. 1997

Brown, Marybeth. Ph.D., P.T., and Kohrt, Wendy. Ph.D.. <u>Endurance Training of the Older Adult</u>. contributor Geriatric Physical Therapy. Mosby-Year Book, Inc. 1993

Brown, Marybeth, Ph.D., P.T. <u>The Well Elderly</u>. contributor. Geriatric Physical Therapy. Mosby-Year Book. 1993

Craik, Rebecca L. Ph. D., P.T. <u>Sensorimotor Changes and Adaptation in the Older Adult</u>. contributor Geriatric Physical Therapy. Mosby-Year Book, Inc. 1993

Dahm, Diane, M.D and Smith, Jay, M.D. <u>Mayo Clinic Fitness for Everybody</u>. Mayo Clinic. Rochester, Minnesota. 2005

Delavier, Frederic. Gundill, Michael. <u>Delavier's Core Anatomy Training</u>. Editions Vigot 2010. Human Kinetics

Ettinger, Walter H., MD, Wright, Brenda S., Ph.D and Blair, Steven N.,PED. <u>Fitness After 50</u> .

Guccione, Andrew A., Ph.D.,P.T. edited by <u>Geriatric Physical Therapy</u>. Mosby-Year Book, Inc.1993 (list of contributing writers, page v and vi)

Kelsey, James. Kinesioligist ARTIC. specialist in SCI and pain. <u>Keltic Hands</u>. A course designed to use acupuncture points in the hands. Taught to US Veterans. 2008

Lewis-McCormick, Irene. <u>The HITT Advantage…High Intensity Workouts for Women</u>. Human Kinetics. 2016

McCall, Pete CSCS, forward by Petersen Gunnar. <u>Ageless Intensity: High-Intensity workout to Slow the Aging Process.</u>. Human Kinetics. 1972

Meyers, Thomas W. <u>Anatomy Trains. Myofacial Meridians for Manual Therapist and Movement Professionals. Elsevier. 2021</u>

Netter, Frank H., MD. <u>Atlas of Human Body</u>. Sixth Edition. Saunders, an imprint of Elsevier, Inc. 2014

Newman, Donald A. <u>Kinesiology of the Musculosketal System</u>, Mosby, Inc. Elseier division. 2010

Page, Phil. Ellenbecker, Todd. <u>Strength Band Training</u> Human Kinetics 2005

Robinson, Lynne and Convy, Gerry. <u>Pilates Workout</u>. Friedman/Fairfax Publishers distributed by Sterling Publishing Company, New York. 2000

Reviewed by Ruth Sova. <u>Fit 'n Fun…Water Exercises for Women (and maybe some men)</u>. offered by Jalkanen Foundation. 2014 especially pages 140;159;164;173;186

Sova, Ruth. <u>Aquatic Exercise</u> second edition. DSL, Ltd. Port Washington. WI. 2000

Belleview Spine and Wellness, Weekly Health Update, assorted articles - Greenwood Village, CO 80111 dchealthupdates.com

Biography

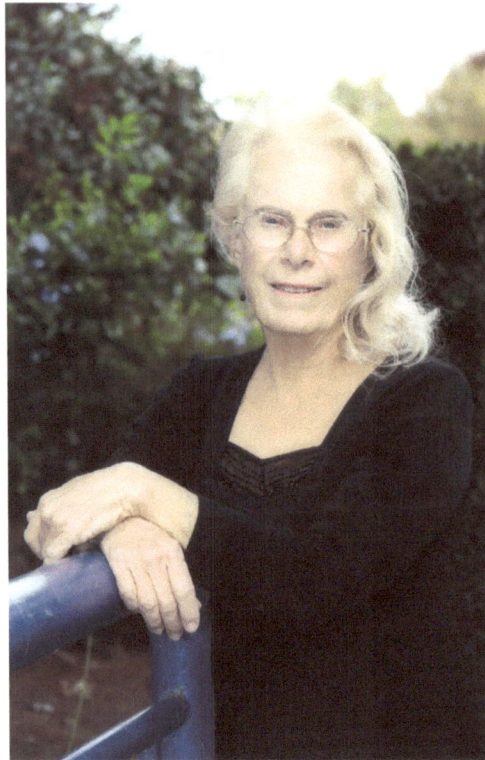

Born in the rural town of Tehachapi, California, Marti Sprinkle, Master of Arts in Organizational Management (MAOM), is a certified water aerobics instructor with over 35 years of experience. She is certified through the American Exercise Association (AEA) and is a member of Aquatic Therapy and Rehabilitation Institute (ATRI). She holds specialty certificates for Total Joint Replacement, Hip and Back, Back-Hab, Aqua Pilates, Integrated Core Training, Rheumatology, and AiChi. AiChi is a water-based relaxation progression designed to increase energy and promote flexibility and muscle strength.

Marti specializes in therapeutic exercises in a commercial spa. Her passion is to better assist her clients as they reach personal health and fitness goals. Marti teaches water aerobics for all ages. Outside of the water, Marti is a concert violinist, performing in several symphonies including solo work. She is the proud mother of a successful daughter, a hiker, and a "parent" of two dogs.

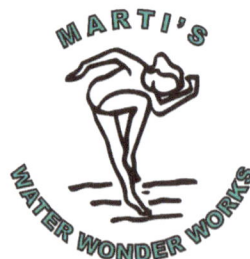

Notes

www.ingramcontent.com/pod-product-compliance
Lightning Source LLC
Chambersburg PA
CBHW060801270326
41926CB00002B/44

* 9 7 8 1 7 7 1 4 3 5 6 0 4 *